A Personal Peace

A Personal Peace

Macrobiotic Reflections On
Mental And Emotional Recovery

David Briscoe
and
Charlotte Mahoney-Briscoe

Japan Publications, Inc.

Note to the reader: Those with health problems are advised to seek the guidance of a qualified medical or psychological professional in addition to a qualified macrobiotic counselor before implementing any of the dietary and other approaches presented in this book. It is essential that any readers who have any reason to suspect serious illness in themselves or their family members seek appropriate medical, nutritional, or psychological advice promptly. Neither this or any other health related book should be used as a substitute for qualified care or treatment.

Published by JAPAN PUBLICATIONS, INC., Tokyo and New York

Distributors:
UNITED STATES: *Kodansha International/USA, Ltd., 114 Fifth Avenue, New York, N. Y. 10011.* CANADA: *Fitzhenry & Whiteside Ltd., 195 Allstate Parkway, Markham, Ontario, L3R 4T8.* MEXICO AND CENTRAL AMERICA: *HARLA S. A. de C. V., Apartado 30–546, Mexico 4, D. F.* BRITISH ISLES: *Premier Book Marketing Ltd., 1 Gower Street, London WC1E 6HA.* EUROPEAN CONTINENT: *European Book Service PBD, Strijkviertel 63, 3454 PK De Meern, The Netherlands.* AUSTRALIA AND NEW ZEALAND: *Bookwise International, 54 Criffendon Road, Findon 5023, South Australia.* THE FAR EAST AND JAPAN: *Japan Publications Trading Co., Ltd., 1–2–1, Sarugaku-cho, Chiyoda-ku, Tokyo 101.*

First edition: May 1989

LCCC No. 88–81757
ISBN 0–87040–698–1

Printed in U.S.A.

To Cindy
>who transforms the day with tenderness and
>feminine strength
>>D. B.

To Vernon
>who has always stood at my side.
>>C. M. B.

>and
For all who suffer in their self-made prisons.

"Every millionth of a second you are changing."
                              —GEORGE OHSAWA

"Listen to the immensity calling."
                              —J. KRISHNAMURTI

"Suffering is the beginning of consciousness."
                              —DOSTOEVSKY

Acknowledgments

My life has been blessed by the presence of extraordinary individuals. This book is as much theirs as mine, for without them I never would have begun this journey.

Unending gratitude goes out to all who have honored me by allowing me to share the precious day with them, especially the following:

Sister Scholastica Schuster, O.S.B., teacher, philosopher, poet, and friend, whose affectionate solidity deeply nourished all who knew her.

J. Krishnamurti, that full flame of humanity, who challenged me with devastating clarity and love to "Wake up!"

Michio Kushi, who invited me to write this book, and whose generosity, friendship, and awesome comprehension of life endlessly inspires me and countless others.

Herman Aihara, the gem of wisdom and wit, whose macrobiotic books and writings ignited my desire to return to writing.

Vernon, my father, the most intelligent man I know, whose justice, fortitude, and equanimity have given each of his five children something great.

My mother, Charlotte, who nurtured me, her once distraught and confused son, long after others would have given up in despair. She gifted me with a love for writing and the urge to discover life beyond the mediocre.

Justin, Nora, Ira, and Iris, my beloved children, who liberated me from the prison of self-obsessed living.

Cindy, best friend, wife, and artist, who designed the cover and illustrations. Her singular intuition guided each page which follows.

DAVID BRISCOE

Contents

Preface

I MAY BE THE FIRST MEDICALLY DIAGNOSED SCHIZOPHRENIC who has recovered as a result of practicing macrobiotics. I won't be the last. What a privilege to be one among many pioneers whose life experience is proving the value of macrobiotics long before science and medicine become enticed by it. It is simply a matter of time until they discover the healing facts of macrobiotics. Here and there they have already begun to take notice.

It is my sincere prayer that macrobiotics is fully understood and practiced as much more than a symptomatic medical approach, though. There is the danger that only its nutritional aspects will be assimilated once their healing benefits are more widely researched and revealed. It would be a shame, indeed a tragedy, if the underlying essence and spirit of macrobiotics were to be brushed aside by the oncoming inevitable absorption of macrobiotic nutritional approaches by the health-care professions.

I have tried to write a book dealing more with the macrobiotic spirit of living. From the beginning I was determined to create a book that would go beyond my own limited story of recovery. Mental health is of great importance to everyone, so I have tried to write a book that embraces each reader. If it challenges you to explore your own life, I will be pleased. Our years are very short here on this earth. Please don't waste your life.

I have not written a book that explores the many different types of mental illness and psychological theories, or how to apply macrobiotic principles to them. For that, another much larger volume will be needed. I have written a personal book based on my own practice and experience. I am not a medical doctor or scientist, so I have not used science and medicine to explain or to validate my recovery and practices.

My mother wrote the first two chapters while recovering from a heart attack. I am grateful for her willingness to return to those years of my youth and remember the agonies.

The rest of the book contains everything I have done until now to discover and uncover the wonders of life. I am happy to pass it on to you.

As I finish these words on a lovely spring morning, there comes silence, and the unmistakable presence of peace.

DAVID BRISCOE

Kansas City, Kansas
April, 1988

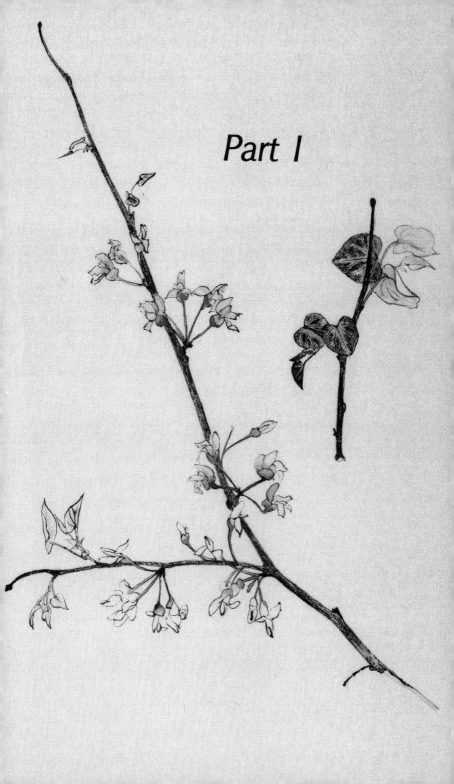

Part I

M Y SON'S PRESENT FRIENDS, ASSOCIATES, AND STUDENTS cannot imagine the kind of person he was in the past. He has evolved through a metamorphosis as drastic as that of caterpillar to butterfly. But in order to know what a person has evolved *from*, one must understand something of the evolution. Therefore, I have written the first two chapters of this book in order to explain David's evolution from that of a mentally ill boy and man into the whole and sane person he is today: husband, father, teacher, businessman, and writer.

I knew his inherent promise before the dark years of mental illness smothered it temporarily. I was his closest and most involved companion during the long, bleak journey before his recovery. I was privy to his misery and pain and fear—and often bore the brunt of those intense emotions.

David asked me to write these chapters, believing that my unique position as both participant and observer would create a viewpoint through which the parents and families of mentally ill patients could discover some harbinger of hope where none had previously existed.

Finally, I must add that David's recovery through the application of macrobiotic principles to his life cannot be proved scientifically. It is, nonetheless, a simple yet astounding truth.

Chapter 1

The Journey Into Mental Illness

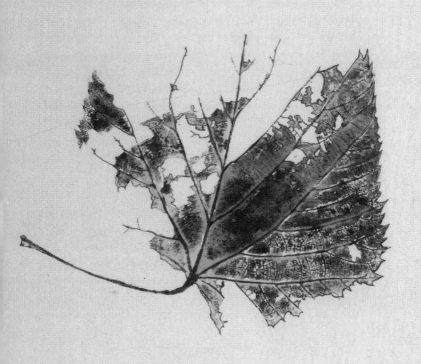

H E MIGHT AS WELL BE DEAD," I kept whispering to myself in the hospital corridor as the heavy doors with wire-reinforced windows swung closed behind our son, David, and the lock ominously thunked into the latchpiece. Even the wire in the window negated him, casting large X's from its criss-cross design onto his back, as if voiding his future.

As far as the society of the sixties was concerned, when David was diagnosed schizophrenic he was the same as dead; condemned to a netherworld of hospitals, medications, whispers, and embarrassment. Schizophrenics and their families had little else to hope for considering the skimpiness of knowledge on the subject during the late sixties and seventies.

At that time many psychotherapists routinely prescribed electroshock therapy, while others dispensed an array of newly created—and not well-understood—psychotropic drugs. Severe schizophrenics were institutionalized, but others, like David, were kept in the mainstream heavily sedated with Stelazine, Thorazine, or both. The diagnosis and definition of schizophrenia was even more of a mystery then than it is today. Diet was never widely considered a major factor either as a cause or as a possible treatment of schizoprehnia and other mental or emotional illnesses. I recently conducted a computer data base search through a university medical library and failed to find any book or periodical of that era in which diet was implicated. It would be many years before the importance of diet could be offered to David and others with similar conditions.

As the nurse led David away to some unknown and frightening destination that morning, we agonized to help him or hold him, but we felt guilty and paralyzed, only capable of handing him over to the care of strangers. Was this place to be his home forever? The glass in the door was like ice between us and our son. Could we ever get through to him? Could he ever break through to us?

The air in the corridor, filled with an almost palpable negative energy whose tendrils hung from the ceiling and walls and crept around our feet, entangled us in a jungle of self-judgments, strangers in white coats, and deep foreboding. As we stared through the wire in the windows, we became conscious of other eyes peering out at us. Some weary, some wild, some·blank, they had come before David, and now they were to be his companions on this journey into a very uncertain future.

The anguish we felt at that moment was hardly a stranger. We had often shared it during the years since David reached pre-adolescence, hoping he would change, only to have our hopes dashed again and again. We had five children, three boys and two girls. All seemed to be healthy and well-adjusted, including David—before he reached the time for passage into puberty. Then I began to sense subtle changes in his personality, a distancing of himself from friends and family, and a reluctance for socializing in general. He became steadily withdrawn and solitary. Life seemed to become an enemy, and his room on the third floor of our home became his fortress against it. Alarmed, I took him for comprehensive testing at one of our local medical centers which had received national acclaim for the quality of its clinic. Every applicable examination was given to David, and the test results indicated that he was perfectly healthy physically and mentally. "Don't worry," the child psychologist said, "I'm sure you'll notice a marked change in your son by the time he reaches puberty."

He was right in his prediction. There was a change—for the worse. He developed an exaggerated appetite for sugar: candy, cookies, and ice cream. At the same time he developed a love for well-done steak and very salty foods like crackers and potato chips. He became fat and hated himself. After eating excessively he would diet excessively. Occasionally he would buy diet drinks and eat nothing until his supply ran out. Some days he would fast totally but would finally return to former habits of excessive eating, especially in secret. The rest of his behavior became characterized by similar obsessiveness, and we tried to convince ourselves that it was simply the usual and temporarily confused adolescent pattern. "It will pass," we predicted. It did not.

His behavior was punctuated with bizarre incidents. Once, he plucked out all of his eyelashes. Another time I found him staring at the cold ashes of a trash fire he had lit hours before. Many years later, he told me about crouching for hours on his hands and knees on a ledge under the basement stairs rather than face the day at school. He would emerge at lunchtime to eat and then return to his hiding place under the stairs when the others went back to school. When we moved to another house, he continued this behavior, sitting quietly and motionlessly in our cold garage until he was sure that the school day was ended. I had no knowledge of these incidents at the time, because students were accepted back into class after an absence upon the presentation of an "excuse note" signed by a parent. David had learned to forge my handwriting.

As a young boy he seemed almost mystically sensitive to anything in his environment—trees, animals, people, conversations. He was able to perceive the spirit of things, and energies and impressions would at times invade his mind in overwhelming torrents. In shops, restaurants, and family gatherings he would be aware of details ignored or unseen by other children and most adults. Later, he would comment on what he saw or felt: the inner qualities of the waitresses, the lonely man in a corner booth, the bitterness in faces—or the laughter. He could sense people's pasts and feel into their futures. Nothing seemed to escape his attention. He was aware and perceptive beyond a boy's emotional capacity to handle the constant barrage of input his mind was receiving.

He developed a passive persona to hide behind and with which he met the world. It seemed impossible to pierce this facade. To his brothers and sisters he was just a loner, and most of his teachers dismissed him as a "shy, average student." Only one or two insightful ones sensed his buried creative talents. Occasionally, at the end of class he would bring his poems or plays to a sensitive teacher, and once or twice he was encouraged to have his plays performed by the class. He loved the acclaim which would bring him out of his shell momentarily. Writing seemed to be a catharsis for him, and the only way he had of expressing his deepest feelings and observations. On special occasions, like Christmas or my birthday, he would delight me with a poem.

One year, when the city fire department was conducting its annual slogan contest, David decided to submit an entry after the small successes of his plays. To his total disbelief, it was announced at a school assembly that he had won the contest. In his shy and intimidated manner he walked across the stage to receive the certificate as the student body collectively giggled and laughed at the fire marshal's jokes about David's clothes being a "few sizes too small for such a fat boy!" He never entered another writing contest.

Because of his passive and reserved nature, David was easy prey for teasers and bullies, especially among the boys, who seemed to take such pleasure in taunting him. To them he was "David Brisket," or "David Crisco," the fat kid. Whispers of "queer," or "fairy" dogged him down the halls. Internally devastated, he'd pretend to be oblivious to the jibes and jeers. Sometimes, though, he'd be stricken with diarrhea or wet his pants out of fear during particularly frightening encounters with classmates.

At home, in his room, it was a different world. It was *his* world, *his* room, *his* sanctuary, and he basked in the freedom and relief that solitude brought. It was here that his true personality would emerge from the locked depths of his mind. He would laugh then, dance, play solitary games, and listen to music. He loved music, movies, and everything gentle and whimsical and tender.

He found all these qualities in one of his aunts, Aunt Bessie. She became the sweet companion of his childhood, never critical or judgmental and always supportive and unconditionally loving. He couldn't wait to spend the weekends with her whenever she would invite him, and they'd spend two days together in her tiny apartment with David cushioned against his fears, doubts, and anxieties. He told me that to him Aunt Bessie's apartment was like a sacred grotto where the world he disliked could not come. Those weekends were safe and solid stepping stones across the painful pond of his childhood. Her death in 1963 was devastating to him because in his mind she was the only person who loved him just as he was.

As he entered high school he developed increasing inconsistencies in his behavior and personality, but he had become so adept at *appearing* to be normal and to fit into our busy family atmosphere, that at first we hardly noticed. Perhaps his abnormal behavior had been present so long that it appeared to be the norm.

He loved the ceremony and competitiveness of high school sporting events, but had a terror of teams and gangs of boys. He secretly admired athletes, but was not athletic himself. In fact, in gym class he was inept, awkward, and uncoordinated. Some days, he said, he would vomit in the rest room before going to gym class, knowing what he would have to face in the way of threats and jokes from the coach and jocks.

Even more than gym, however, he dreaded the speech class. Oral reports reduced him to a twitching insomniac days before they were scheduled, but he would inevitably find the courage to face the terror-filled moment and survive it. Strange, that as his horror of public speaking grew worse, his love of performing as an actor grew more intense. Any play or musical in which he could win a role allowed him to be seen as someone other than the unlikable and repulsive person he perceived himself to be.

Sometimes he would shock us with extreme displays of self-assertion and extroversion, and at other times he would be so depressed and withdrawn that it seemed all the energy and color had been drained from him. Once he announced he had found a job at a local record store, and we were stunned but overjoyed at this attempt at maturity, only to watch him become physically ill from worry each day before he was scheduled to report for work. He quit within two weeks of starting.

As he progressed through high school David seemed to become physically ill more often. He was hospitalized with an acute kidney problem. He developed sore throats, fevers, and digestive problems in increasing numbers. When he reached his senior year he was hospitalized with a duodenal ulcer. He had been on the razor's edge too long. We decided he should be seen by a psychiatrist while he was in the hospital.

At the time, there was a heavy stigma attached to mental illness and psychiatry. David didn't seem to mind, however. In fact, he developed an attachment to the world of the hospital, nurses, and doctors. The secure, controlled atmosphere and the attention showered on his physical well-being delighted him. He discovered that illness could be a tool for avoiding the encroaching realities and responsibilities of what he considered to be a harsh world lying in wait for him after graduation.

To David, it *was* an incredibly harsh world. The childhood that he had extended many years longer than most young people of his age was now truly over. His best friend of many years had moved away and David felt completely lost. He plunged deeply into depression, and began what was to become a six-year saga of psychiatric sessions and a miserable partnership with a pill, the newly created drug, Thorazine. At best, it allowed him to function minimally. The results of further tests caused our doctors to paint an ugly picture of David's capabilities, invoking in our minds the future scenario of an aging son submerged in medication and supervised by guardians. We were advised not to entertain any thoughts of college or any kind of long-term relationships where David was concerned. "His mind," they said, "is too distorted and chaotic to concentrate on anything." The void between David's inner world of imagination, fears, and anxieties, and the external world presented too wide a gap for him to bridge.

That summer of 1967, now a famous one in the history of

American sociology, almost spelled the end of David's life. It was the era of flower children, hippies, LSD, marijuana and other drugs, rejecting parents and their lifestyle, and running away from home. It was also the era of the Beatles, and David had been obsessed with their music for several years. He would often lie in his room for hours listening to their newest single. Once, when their latest album was released, he walked for two miles in a blizzard to buy it. In the summer of '67, *Sgt. Pepper's Lonely Hearts Club Band* was released. It was purported to be filled with songs having numerous references to drugs, "dropping out," and leaving home. His mind on fire with frustration, David was infatuated with the rebellious ideas. He was certain that the hippies would be sympathetic pals who would welcome his strange ideas, visions, and idiosyncrasies.

After working part-time at a job which he thoroughly detested, David secretly saved enough money to buy a round-trip ticket to San Francisco whose Haight-Ashbury district had been widely publicized as the mecca of flower children and hippies. Later, he told us that he was not running away from home, but only planning to take what he thought would be a challenging and exciting trip. He didn't realize that life among the "gentle" hippies could be a harsher and more dangerous one than he'd ever dreamed of, and that with that bus ticket he would have bought his way into a nightmare world of opportunists, robbers, and potential murderers.

He didn't even have to go all the way to San Francisco to meet his first hippie "pal." He boarded the bus at Kansas City, and was immediately appealing to David because with his strange-looking clothes and long hair he epitomized the perfect hippie. After many of the passengers disembarked along the way, the young hippie introduced himself and they rode the rest of the way together. It was to prove an introduction to terror.

In Reno, Nevada, David's new-found buddy left the bus, returning with two paper bags. From a small suitcase he extracted a tube of airplane glue from a supply of about two dozen he carried. He squirted some into one of the bags and demonstrated how to place it over the nose and mouth, and breathe the fumes deeply. David was "high" for the first time. What a combination—our naive son's uncontrolled imagination and mind-expanding drugs!

David and his compatriot arrived in San Francisco one morning searching for an address given by another "pal" where both of them would be welcome to stay. David retched constantly as they walked in and out of dingy doorways and hangouts of his new friend. He had also confided to his pal that he kept his money inside his sock, so that by the time they found the address and were welcomed inside by two girls who seemed to live there, the plan must have already been underway to separate David from his possessions. For some reason it didn't go into effect immediately because he recalls being there a day or two, smoking marijuana, and eating very little. Although he doesn't remember it, he must have ingested some kind of hallucinatory drug also, because he lost consciousness at a party to which his friends escorted him.

When he regained consciousness, he was groping his way through Golden Gate Park, apparently having been dumped there the night before. He had no money, no shoes, no bus ticket, no luggage, and definitely not any friends. He had no memory of the party except the dim recall of being approached with a sexual proposition from one of his pal's buddies. There were many transients in the park, including one insistent individual who kept threatening him with a gun unless he'd agree to come with him. As David attempted to cope with this new nightmare, a young couple riding by recognized his distress, disengaged him somehow from the wild-acting stranger, and delivered him to the Haight-Ashbury Free Clinic. He was surrounded by screaming youngsters on bad "trips," and others who had overdosed. But he was alive and could get professional help there. The young Samaritans had probably saved his life.

Meanwhile, during David's absence we were barely functioning as a family. We, his parents, were grief-stricken at not being able to bring our son home from wherever he was. His brothers and sisters were quiet and apprehensive. His vacant place at the table cast a pall over all of us. We were a splintered group. One of us was missing.

Finally, after several days and nights of anguished waiting, the phone rang, and a calm, assured voice said, "Shalom, Mrs. Briscoe. I have news of your son." It was the medical doctor from the Free Clinic informing me that David had been taken by the police to the junior psychiatric and security ward of a nearby hospital. I thanked him effusively, and as early as possible the next day I contacted the hospital and told them I would be out on the next flight. When I arrived, the staff seemed amazed that I had appeared so soon. It was evident that few parents were eager to reclaim their wayward children.

When they brought David to see me he appeared dazed and disoriented. He hardly responded to my questions, and I'm not sure he even recognized me. It was as if he now existed in some strange new dimension which I could never hope to enter and share. I remained in the city several days, visiting David at the hospital while psychiatric chaperones supervised our meetings. They finally agreed to allow David to return to Kansas City with me.

We boarded the plane without incident although the staff psychiatrist had warned me to watch for some kind of reaction, even though David was heavily sedated. After a dreadful trip in which I had to remain constantly alert for any sudden movement from my son, we landed in Kansas City and were met by his grave and apprehensive father. David's psychiatrist wanted us to take him directly to the psychiatric ward of St. Mary's Hospital as soon as we arrived. After consulting David so that he would realize we wanted to be fair with him and allow him a choice, we drove him to the hospital at 5:30 in the morning and admitted him.

After weeks of private therapy and trials with different medications, David was released into our care and allowed to return home. We wondered how he would function in the future when we were no longer there to care for him. Many, many uncertainties burned inside us at the end of the summer of 1967.

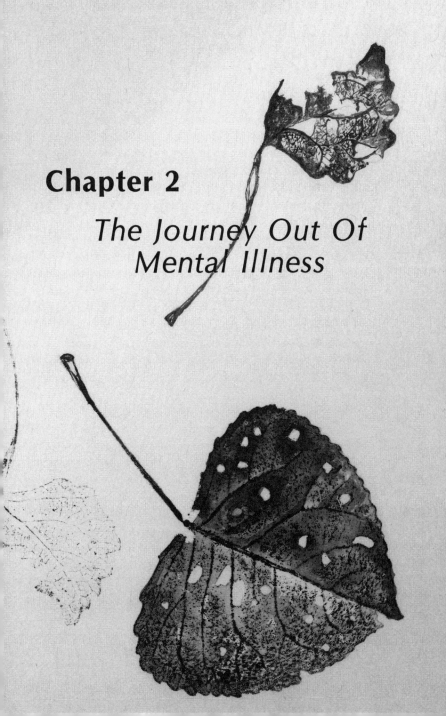

Chapter 2

The Journey Out Of Mental Illness

> I am today
> As I was the day
> Of my birth—
> Never more
> Never less
> Forever becoming
> What I have always been.

I ENCOURAGED OUR CHILDREN to give us something of themselves for Christmas, so the above poem was David's Christmas gift to me the winter of 1967. I restrained the sob in my throat until he left the room. It seemed a forlorn, fatalistic piece which only reiterated the medical prognosis that his mental condition would never change. Christmas can make us joyous and uplifted or vulnerable to depression—even desolation. That Christmas was the first one on which I had to face the seemingly irrefutable fact that our son would always be a schizophrenic. His poem only gave emphasis to my feeling of desolation.

Which of us was capable of recognizing this poem as the muffled plea from David's soul as it cried out for recognition from beneath suffocating layers of medication in a body already chemically imbalanced? Not David, surely, who was still jousting with his private devils, and certainly not I who had already lit too many candles of hope only to watch them being snuffed out one by one as each new crisis arrived. I didn't realize that we had lit a candle of hope whose flame would never be snuffed out, when we agreed to let David register at a local private junior college in spite of the results of psychological testing which stamped him as mentally unfit for college. Besides that, a mind as unstable as David's had been in the past, coupled with whatever damage he may have sustained from his San Francisco fiasco, persuaded the psychiatrist and us to believe that attending college would at the most be therapeutic for David, and at the very least a time filler.

What force guides one to make proper or inappropriate

choices? Whose hands offer the lantern to the lost ones so that
its beam can illuminate the dark labyrinths of life? We thought
we had helped David. Now we know that God was the moving force, because each step that David took from this point
onward propelled him toward a rebirth.

The first step was into a composition class taught by Sister
Scholastica Schuster, O.S.B., a master teacher. In David's case
she was a teacher/healer and he learned to love her dearly.
She began the long process of healing which would grind
a deep, exhausting trail across our lives for the next seven
years by tucking him under her wing, and spending many
hours of her precious time listening to him, counseling him,
and encouraging him to stretch his mind beyond himself.
She helped him calm the chaos of his mind periodically with
tranquil trips into the world of the great writers and poets,
some of whom had suffered from mental problems more
severe than David's. Eventually, Sister Scholastica wrote
a college textbook on creative writing which was published
by Random House and which contains two of David's poems.
He would have been happy staying there forever, but she
encouraged him to move on.

It seemed impossible to us that David could actually have
completed two years of college and had been accepted at one
of our state universities. In retrospect, I realize he was being
buoyed up and moved along by some protective current of
divine origin. We were happy but naive, thinking that he
could move into an apartment with his older brother who
attended the same university, and that it would be a stabiliz-
ing factor in his life. With his own difficult curriculum and
part-time job, David's brother scarcely had time for more than
a cursory evaluation of David's outward demeanor.

His normal outward behavior masked so much inner
turmoil, but his major in theater and his acting talent helped
David hide his ever-present paranoia from his brother and
his own friends. They didn't know he had a constant voice
in his head that was so ever-present he thought it was a
normal condition of everyone's mind. They weren't aware

that when he walked into a room he thought everyone was looking at *him*, talking about *him*; nor that he was so extremely sensitive to his environment that he was aware of auras of hidden feelings in the room, sensing people's thoughts, or having strong premonitions about those who were present. They wouldn't have believed that nice, normal David often walked the streets of the university town late at night, drugged and disoriented, not knowing who or where he was. Nor could they have believed that he missed so many classes because he had taken asylum under his bedcovers each of those days, totally concealing himself from the terrors that threatened him.

He usually managed to cope with his personal terrors through daily intake of Thorazine and monthly or bi-monthly visits to the psychiatrist. When he was home, I could monitor his dosage of Thorazine, but back at college, in his confused mental state, he would often take three tablets three times a day rather than the proper *one* tablet three times a day. When he had taken an overdose, he would call me, whimpering disconnected phrases in a slurred voice about being desperate and lonely. I would be frantic and frustrated that I could do so little to help him via long distance other than warn again and again that he must be constantly aware of the danger of over-medication. Of course we had an option: we could always have demanded that he drop out of college and return home, but that would have meant the death of hope for David and for us.

Hope. It was a scarce commodity in the sixties and seventies for schizophrenics and their families. There seemed to be no new developments in the cause or treatment of schizophrenia. It was still generally accepted by the medical community and society at large that the home environment was directly responsible for the illness, either through parents withholding love and attention or from their too rigid discipline. Those of us who were parents of schizophrenics shared a universal sense of overpowering guilt, besides becoming quite skillful in adroitly fielding questions about the nature of our children's illness, except to our families and close friends.

I admit to the guilt of being abusively passive in my attitude toward David's diet. I prepared nutritionally balanced meals but I seldom served a formal dessert, so I considered David's obsession with concentrated forms of sugar to be just a natural craving. The cry of alarm had not yet been sounded about the havoc which sugar could wreak on the mind and body, nor about the harm of additives in food. My generation could be said to have "buried their heads in the sand," except that the quote is usually attributed to something unpleasant or threatening. We didn't connect either of these adjectives to sugar.

Apparently, desserts were less plentiful at school because David would go on a sugar binge when he was home on a break or for a visit to the psychiatrist. We always had ice cream in the freezer, for instance, and one of his favorite desserts was a large bowl of vanilla ice cream smothered with brown sugar. As a result of this kind of binge, we would ride the roller-coaster of his violent mood changes, rising to the top then plunging to the depths. Yes, the thought occurred to me that he was eating too much sugar, but it never occurred to me that the sugar might be causing his mood changes.

I suffered his caustic moods as long as I could, hoping that it might help him purge his soul of whatever kind of devil had taken up residence there. But I could never find it in my heart to say that he was "not guilty by reason of insanity," because I never believed him insane. I felt that he had to be held responsible for his actions and his words, so I was never all martyr nor a constantly loving mother during his verbal attacks. I was human, I bled, and when struck in a vulnerable spot, defended myself. I would search his eyes after these confrontations to see if they were free of the lost, wild look, but it always hid there furtively and elusively in their depths.

After he had emptied himself of the raving and closed himself up in his room, I would listen at his door for some sound, some movement, terrified that he would finally embrace the idea that he could only find personal peace in suicide. I had often found crumpled notes on his desk which lent credence to my fear. I kept searching for *some* means of making his life and ours more bearable, but there were simply no options available except for institutionalizing or the constant medication and dependence on the psychiatrist. Bills from the pharmacy and the psychiatrist represented a terrible financial drain, but that was the option we chose. It became a normal way of life, without change, and without hope.

One small glimmer of hope appeared his senior year at college, shining upward through a pile of paperback books left outside his door by a friend. We wouldn't have recognized the light if we had seen it, and it only attracted David's attention because of its title, *Zen Macrobiotic Cooking* by Michel Abesehra. At the time, he was intrigued by Oriental cultures and religions, and after quickly riffling through its pages, went out in search of a health-food store. Although it was woefully inadequate in everything except vitamins, it did have a box of brown rice and a bottle of tamari, the shelf life of which had long ago expired. He remembered both as required items for a recipe in the cookbook and bought them in anticipation of his first venture in macrobiotic cooking. When his first attempt produced a pathetic pan of underdone rice swimming in ancient tamari, he lost interest in macrobiotics, the cookbook was left to languish on the shelf, and he returned to his former diet.

At that time there were no macrobiotic cooking classes available in the university area. In fact, even *knowledge* of the word was limited to a small esoteric group who were simply dipping their toes into anything sounding exotic. Then, when David returned home after miraculously graduating with a degree in theater, he forgot macrobiotics altogether because it enjoyed even less publicity in our small town than it had in the more adventurous climate of the university community.

He fell into a deep depression after being rejected by VISTA and the draft. Strangely enough, if he had been accepted by the Army he would have resented it, but having to face the reality that neither organization was interested in having those with a history of mental illness reduced him to a state of melancholy. He managed to rouse himself from this state after reading an ad in our local newspaper inviting people to a "Class in Macrobiotic Cooking." His decision took a great deal of courage because he knew he'd be faced with the emotional stress of meeting strange new people who might prove too challenging for his mind.

Macrobiotic! What a strange, scientific-sounding word for a cooking class. That, at the least, seemed to be the consensus of the local media. It engendered so much interest within the TV news media that one station sent a crew to film the first class. What a pity that we don't have a tape of the event because it marked the time of David's rebirth.

The young woman who taught the class was quite knowledgeable about macrobiotics, and she cooked delicious food which transcended David's original rice-tamari dish. He seemed to know from that day that he was irrevocably committed to macrobiotics, not because of any premonition that he would be healed but because he felt deeply that the foods were more healthful and beneficial to a person's whole life. Neither he nor we realized at the time that anything so simple could create a strong healing process, nor that the healing process was already underway.

Meanwhile, he made a few new friends from among the members of the cooking class and began to wean himself from us with the help of various jobs which paid enough to support him in a small apartment. He was still committed to Thorazine and the psychiatrist, however.

What a jumble his life was at that time! At one period he was a houseboy, at another he was a custodian in a school. Both jobs were really escape hatches from life. Both provided anonymity and isolation. In one sense he was moving ahead. In another he was on a treadmill going nowhere.

When David's psychiatrist informed us he was leaving his practice and going to another state where he thought it might be more beneficial to his own children's mental health, I believe I felt more anxiety and agitation than David. His

mental equilibrium still remained fragile, and I was fearful
that he might be completely unbalanced by this disastrous new
However, he seemed to take it in stride while I felt abandoned
and unable to wrestle with David's mental problems without
professional help. I was unimpressed that his psychiatrist was
uprooting himself from a lucrative practice and moving his
family to an area which could boast, at least statistically, of
possessing a healthier moral climate in which to raise children.
I also envied his ability and freedom to leave.

We were lucky to be able to make immediate arrangements
with a young psychologist who had been recommended by
our doctor, and he seemed able to establish immediate
rapport with David. During this time of uncertainty David
was doing everything within his power to stay with macrobiotics and not revert to his old, disabling diet, and I must add
receiving little support from me in his "weird way of eating."

It seemed that only a short time had passed when he informed us that he was planning to discontinue his visits to the
psychologist as well as his constant use of Thorazine. He
planned, he said, from that moment on, to take control of his
mental and physical health, and in effect to heal himself. We
thought it was a dangerous decision but we were unable to
convince him differently. He discovered that it *was* dangerous
to attempt discontinuing Thorazine abruptly, so he modified
the dosage to a sensible quantity which he was eventually able
to discontinue. Now, instead of wasting his days, he began to
make plans for the future.

He found a job and worked at it long enough to save money
for a trip to California where he studied under, and assisted,
a macrobiotic expert in Oriental teas. He returned home and
again saved money from a job to move to a different area in
California where he attended seminars on macrobiotics and
cooking classes. On his next homecoming his father and I
were shocked at his appearance. We had been foolish enough
to light another candle of hope as a result of David's slowly
developing metamorphosis. Now he looked as if he might be
deliberately starving himself to death. He had deeply hollowed

heeks and his body was without definition; cadaverous. As we
velcomed him home and listened to his experiences I watched
is eyes—my barometer of his sanity—and could see that the
nad look had dissipated to a misty residue like ground fog
uffled by a warm breeze.

Today I believe that he had been following a macrobiotic
iet and a macrobiotic way of life long enough that internal
ehabilitation was taking place as the drugs and chemicals he
ad been involved in so long were being purged from his
ody. Macrobiotics, in effect, was restructuring his body
hemistry into a totally contrasting formula. Along with the
hysical reformation, one could sense the emergence of a
ational, warm and amiable personality.

Proof of the changing personality was a new feeling of ease
e displayed in his relations with young women. Slowly, his
ld feelings of inadequacy and inferiority seemed to disappear.
lmost too quickly, though, he announced plans to marry.
Ve were startled at this announcement because we believed
im far from ready to accept the stresses of marriage, yet we
ould hardly prohibit the wedding of two people over twenty-
ne who were both reasonably aware that stresses could occur.

Although this marriage eventually ended in divorce, it
reated a fine son. In the new role of father, David's life
teadily took on a deeper meaning. As a father he felt he
ould no longer drift from job to job, and as the theater no
onger seemed to attract him after graduation, he decided to
eturn to school and seek a degree in education.

It seemed that each step he took on the journey toward
ealing himself grew longer and more difficult. He took giant
teps in those days, studying, practice-teaching, and working
t a part-time job to support his family. Some days, going to
ork or going to teach must have been as difficult for him as
alking across hot coals. Some days, he didn't make it to
ither place, but stayed home shaking under the bedcovers.
hrough all the crises, however, he continued to eat macro-
iotically.

He persevered in attaining his B.S. in Education, but this

time around his grades were mainly A's rather than his former barely passing ones. He was offered an excellent teaching position in the high school where he was a practicing teacher, but elected to employ his teaching expertise in macro-biotics where he could reach young people like the one he had formerly been, and indeed, people of all ages who had physical or mental problems. I cannot help but remind the readers of this book that we are still referring to the same young man who had been diagnosed by psychiatrists and psychologists as paranoid schizophrenic and who had lived a terror-stricken, mentally chaotic life for fifteen years. This same young man, originally adjudged unfit for college was now the possessor of two college degrees!

The metamorphosis of David seemed to take a cruel length of time, but time isn't relative in reference to the miracle of David's return to us as he was always meant to be. The same spiritual force that had taken his hand and led him through the labyrinthine passages of his life must have also contributed to David's conviction that macrobiotics would be his salvation. Medical personnel might propose different reasons for David's transformation, but my husband and I know it was caused by his macrobiotic diet and way of life, and that he found this answer through God's help. There is no other answer. God was on one side of David, guiding. We were on David's other side, witnessing.

For so many years there were starts and stops and new beginnings; starts and stops and new beginnings once more as David floundered around during his search, and before he stumbled into macrobiotics. Today, others are luckier because there are so many more instructors, seminars, cooking classes and macrobiotic foods available wherever health-conscious people exist.

In writing this book, David hopes to expose more people to the incredible healing benefits of macrobiotics. There are certainly more serious forms of mental illness among the world population, just as there are more serious cases of measles, chicken-pox, and the flu. Some types of mental illness might

not respond to a treatment of macrobiotics and certainly not
to an immature or incomplete practice of it. Proper macrobiotic education is essential. Many patients and their families
might not have the patience that David had. Some will find it
impossible to believe that a simple method could effect such a
recovery: *Diet* can relieve mental illness? I hope that psychiatrists and nutritionists will join forces soon in order to examine
the possibilities of creating mental health through proper
nutrition.

Besides learning about the healing powers of good nutrition,
in David's long journey into and out of mental illness he discovered many facets of macrobiotic living that contributed to
his developing personal peace, and he shares that discovery in
the chapters that follow.

David and his present wife, Cindy, founded a nucleus macrobiotic community in Kansas City. Together they operate the
Amber Waves Cafe and the Macrobiotic Center of Kansas City
where they teach cooking classes, and continue to cook delicious
meals in the cafe for an increasing number of health-conscious
people. David is now a Kushi Institute certified macrobiotic
teacher and counselor. He hopes that you will read this book
and become a participant in the extraordinary adventure of
life.

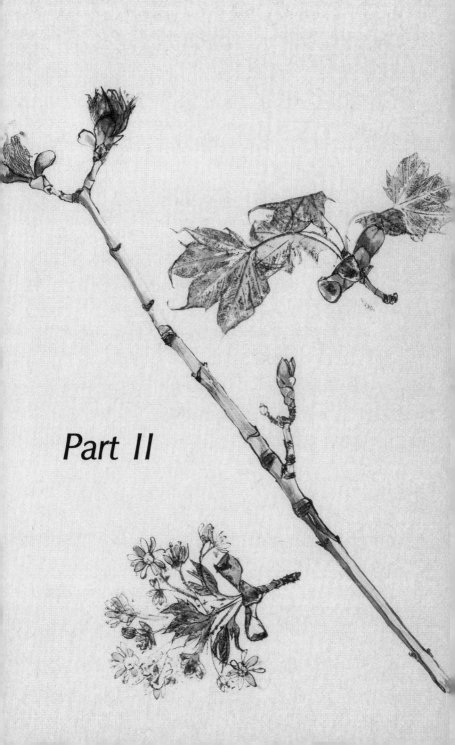

Part II

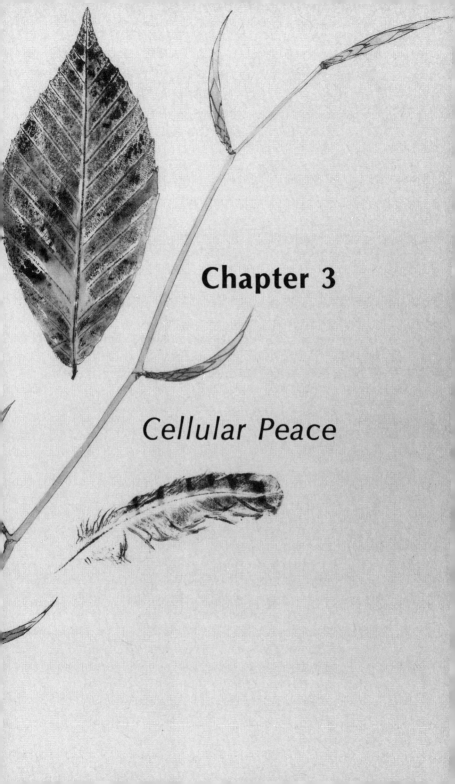

Chapter 3

Cellular Peace

CELLULAR PEACE IS THE FOUNDATION of personal peace. Without it, most attempts to find peace, tranquility, and harmony will end up a futile struggle. There are many who obtain a temporary peace of mind through taking a vacation, changing jobs, entering a new relationship, joining a different religion, and so on, but the ups and downs of daily living erodes this kind of peace after awhile. Without peace in the very cells of your body, life easily becomes a battlefield filled with aches, pains, chronic illness and degenerative disease. Sick people often have a more difficult time making personal peace and peace with the world at large.

What is cellular peace? How does it come about and how can we maintain it? It is surprisingly simple to understand. The application of it changed the course of my entire life. It could do the same for you, if you want.

The vocabulary of cellular peace is made up of three words, basically. They are *energy*, *consumption*, and *elimination*. There are two basic principles of cellular peace. They are as follows:

1. *Everything that you consume must also be eliminated.*
2. *The quality of the energy eliminated will be determined by the quality of the energy consumed.*

These are the most important facts I have learned about the body, cells, organs and their functions, and their relationship to our mental and emotional health. Macrobiotic physiology and the study of its relationship to the level of consciousness is based on these principles.

Modern physics has confirmed the ancient notion that everything is energy. Material phenomena are condensed energy which change slowly enough to appear stable to our eyes. They seem to be permanent because they are visible, but in fact are changing constantly at the cellular level. Other phenomena like gas and sound waves are very expanded forms of energy and so are not visible. Energy in all its endless manifestations and qualities is the stuff of life. Macrobiotics, which is the understanding of energy, is the study of life.

Our food is energy and so is water. Usually, when there is discussion of food, most of us immediately think of the food which we take through our mouths. But there are many other forms of nourishment as well. Of course, we must have the energy provided by protein, carbohydrates, fats, vitamins, and minerals. Without them our lives could not develop, but what are the other types of energy which nurture us? *Everything* that we take into ourselves is energy nourishment; that is, it becomes part of us by entering us, and remains with us until it is eliminated. It can stay with us for just a short time or it might stay much longer, depending on the kind of energy it is and our own physical condition.

The following outline shows the most basic types of energy and where we take them in:

Types of Energy Consumption

Energy	Where Taken In
food and water	mouth
gases (oxygen, etc.)	nose
sound waves	ears
light waves	eyes
heat, cold, pressure	skin surface (nerves)
cosmic waves	brain

We are constantly consuming these various forms of energy. Some we must take regularly or else we would die. Others can be temporarily avoided but soon must be consumed again to avoid serious bodily harm.

Everything we have eaten, inhaled, heard, seen, touched, and felt has been food for us. This has included TV, radio, music, books, ideas, environment, atmosphere, and geographical location. What our teachers have told us, all of the words that our parents spoke to us, their attitude, the home environment of childhood, the lives of our ancestors, and our brothers' and sisters' lives have nourished us, too. Think of all the varieties of energy we have consumed and continue to take daily. It's amazing!

The various qualities of the different kinds of energy can be generally classified into two opposite categories. For example, sound waves can be loud crashing sounds such as those found in cities, rock music, screaming and angry people, or they can be the soft sounds of chamber music, the tranquil sounds of a quiet path in the woods, or the affectionate whispers of a loved one. The external atmosphere can be highly charged and activated by the energy from a bright sun on a clear day, or it can be still, cold, and heavy with the feeling of oppressiveness on a dark and overcast day. The movies that we watch sometimes have beautiful natural scenes, or they can have images of violence and bloodshed. Some parents impart through their behavior the impression that life is enjoyable, and that care, affection and love are essential elements of a happy life. Others impress their children with a philosophy of greed, suspicion, and self-worth based on the amount of money or power one can accumulate.

The food and drink we take through our mouths can have overstimulating effects on the nervous system, or clog the arteries and dull the brain, while others help to maintain normal blood sugar levels and are easily eliminated from the system.

The different qualities of energy that we consume are directly responsible for the quality of energy that we eliminate. Following are the major ways we have for using and eliminating energy:

Ways of Eliminating Energy

Physical	Psychological
Bowel movement	Expressions: Speaking,
Urination	Writing, Art, Ideas
Exhalation	Emotions
Perspiration	Thinking
Exercise	Dreams
Movement	
Gestures	
Speaking	
Cellular activity	

We can say that *everything which comes out of us is an elimination of energy*, for without energy we can't move, think, or speak. We must take in energy in order to fuel the various physiological functions and psychological activities of daily life. If the energy we consume is wild, chaotic, harsh, or violent, the elimination of that energy will be similar. This is an inescapable law of life. When someone manifests symptoms of illness, exhibits bizarre behavior or thinking, we are simply seeing the outward elimination of some of their inwardly, imbalanced energy. When the quality of the energy being consumed is changed, the manifestations of the energy in elimination will also change.

Generally, energy can be categorized into two basic and broad categories: expansive (yin) and contractive (yang). When we learn to so categorize energy, we can better grasp the ideas about their qualities and effects on us. It will be helpful to display the general range between expansive and contractive qualities. In order to make it clear, let's use food as an example. On one end of the spectrum we'll place those foods whose energy is generally most contractive because they are very condensed forms of animal protein, fat, and sodium, or because, due to their cooking and preparation, they have become salty, hard and dry (see chart on the following page).

The most contracting (yang) foods are eggs, beef, pork, chicken and hard cheese. Because animals eat an enormous amount of feed in order to live and grow, this energy becomes highly concentrated in their muscle and fat. When we eat this kind of extremely concentrated energy, strong contracted energy is imparted to our own body cells, functions, activity, behavior, gestures, speaking, etc.

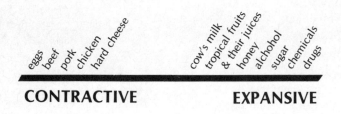

CONTRACTIVE   **EXPANSIVE**

On the other end of the spectrum are the opposite kinds of food containing the expanded (yin) type of energy. Their regular consumption will impart extremely expanding, and therefore, extremely loosening qualities to the body and mentality. They include mind-expanding drugs and chemicals, sugar, alcohol, honey, tropical fruit juices and cow's milk. Most of the foods on the contractive end of the spectrum are high in saturated fats, concentrated protein, salt and cholesterol. Many of the foods on the expansive end are excessively high in refined carbohydrates or potassium.

When we take foods from one end, we automatically desire those from the opposite end. Watch your own way of eating to test this and see if it is so. When we become tense, tight, edgy and irritable due to our inability to adequately use and eliminate the foods with contracting energy, we become intensely attracted to those foods and energies which provide a temporary release or sense of relaxation because of their extremely expansive nature. Such strong release is provided by the energy of alcohol, drugs, sugar and overeating.

When we consume foods which over-relax us, make us physically de-energized and passive, we eventually crave the stimulation provided by the burning energy of animal fat and

cholesterol-rich foods. Nutritionally, we crave refined carbohydrates in order to balance the consumption of concentrated
animal protein and fat. It is a precarious balance at best. This
is the nutritional basis for alcoholism, drug addiction and the
gain-weight/lose-weight cycle of most chronic dieters.

Along with the food's energy contribution to an overly
tight or overly expanded condition within the body and
mentality, there are other contributing factors. When we live
in crowded cities, work under great pressure, become com-
pressed by expectations and responsibilities, or are dogged by
bad memories and nagging thoughts, we are also affected by
yang, pressurizing types of energy that eventually make us
crave quick release and relaxation. We are driven to escape
from this intense pressure, and naturally we are attracted to
the opposite extreme.

The kind of entertainment, relationships, vacations, and
experiences that we choose will reflect the kind of condition we have created in ourselves through eating and daily
living. We are constantly striving for harmony and peace,
even if it is one built of extremes. Extremes of energy, however, never create true harmony because they are too unstable.
What they do create, though, is an uncomfortable and unhealthy seesaw effect on one's physical, mental and emotional
state. One day you are up, the next day down; one day very
confident, the next self-conscious, nervous and shy; one week
you are bursting with physical vitality, the next exhausted
and lagging behind.

When you live on the edge of extremes, your body gets
easily overstimulated, overworked and exhausted. Exercise
addicts are perfect examples of this. Because of the overload of
energy in their systems, they become literally addicted to
jogging, swimming, or some other sport, in an attempt to
eliminate through exercise the excess energy backed up inside
them. If they miss their exercise for very long, they feel
miserable because of the constriction and fatigue caused by
this concentrated energy. Many of these people are killing
themselves through extreme physical overexertion. If they

could learn to reduce the excess internal energy through proper understanding of diet and lifestyle, they could enjoy a normal exercise program without the addiction.

There was a time when people very easily eliminated what they consumed because of a healthier diet and lifestyle. A diet low in animal fats, cholesterol, refined sugar, and high in whole grains and vegetables once created a very healthy human being. Now, only a small minority have whole grains and vegetables as the center of their diet.

I meet many people who think they can sidestep nature's laws by taking food supplements, herbs, fasting, and working out. I can tell you that these people are getting cancer, heart disease, AIDS, diabetes, allergies, and emotional problems just like the rest of society. Because they do not change their daily food consumption, excess builds up in them just like in everyone else. Many of them have come to see me. Professional dietitians, medical doctors, nurses, weight lifters, health-food store owners, jogging champions, holistic-health experts, all develop serious health problems because of their ignorance of the laws of nature and the way of cellular peace. They are astounded to learn of its simplicity.

According to a recent television program, the USDA has released figures that could explain why our consumption and elimination have become extremely out of balance. These figures show that the per-capita consumption of beef in this country now exceeds 150 pounds, milk products comprise over 300 pounds of a person's annual food consumption, soft drinks are contributing 40 gallons of chemicals to each American every year, and sugar consumption is high on the list of excesses with more than 110 pounds being consumed yearly by each person. Chemicals, food additives, preservatives, and colorings add about 14 pounds of sludge to our system yearly. The list goes on and on. Where does all of this energy go? It doesn't just evaporate.

Our body is truly an incredible miracle! It provides everything necessary for a healthy, active, sensitive, and creative approach to life, but the body's physical capacity is limited, and though we may think that we can do whatever we like, eat whatever we like, the truth is we can't. Sure, we can freely consume anything, but the body can only deal with so much. Organically, we have four major areas of elimination: the bowels, kidneys, lungs, and skin. They function marvelously well when they are healthy, but in today's world the majority of people don't have such healthy organs of elimination.

The majority of health problems arise because of weak and ineffective organs of elimination. Our organs make a valiant effort to do their various jobs, but when we continue to overwhelm them with the extra work necessary to deal with our excess consumption, they begin to break down. They never get a rest even when they are exhausted and overworked, unless we change our way of eating. Daily, the onslaught of animal fats and protein, sugar, chemicals, and other food substances flood the body and demand to be eliminated. If waste products are not eliminated, they create a slow poisoning and polluting of the system.

Our body gives us signals that it has become overworked. When you become physically exhausted, you are unable to perform properly, your coordination is impaired, and you can make mistakes. Your organs, being part of you, are no different. What are these signals being given off by the organs alerting us to their exhaustion? If we could learn to recognize them, we might be able to avert serious health problems.

Chronic diarrhea or constipation is a result of overworked and weakened intestines, as is a bad-smelling bowel movement. Bloated abdomens can be seen on many people, especially the elderly and overweight. This often indicates swollen and loose intestines. Overtaxed and tired kidneys create frequent urination (five or more times per day) and chronic night-time urination (urination during the night is not normal).

Most dry skin is caused by blocked pores. Some of the concentrated waste products coming to the surface of the skin gets blocked underneath, and the surface of the skin cannot be properly moisturized. Lungs, burdened by the chronic congestion caused by the consumption of mucus-forming foods, can't properly absorb oxygen nor can they adequately eliminate waste products. Yearly respiratory problems are one sign of overworked lungs.

Though our body gives us these signals, we more often than not continue to shove mouthfuls of fat, sugar, chemicals and cholesterol at the organs every day. Even many health-food enthusiasts and so-called vegetarians advocate the use of high-fat and cholesterol-loaded foods such as eggs, cheese, organic beef, as well as honey and other forms of concentrated sugar. This energy overload cannot be normally eliminated. It forces the organs to fight for their lives, battle for adequate blood supply, fend for themselves at the expense of other organs and inter-organ harmony, resulting in a physiological free-for-all and organic anarchy leading ultimately to that cellular war we call disease.

If you continue to eat the typical American diet, and you haven't suffered from some form of chronic illness by the time you are seventy, write to me and I'll send you congratulations. Only the few who were given astonishingly strong constitutions by their parents evade the eroding effects of the daily American diet.

When our organs can no longer naturally and adequately eliminate, the accumulation of excess energy and matter in the body accelerates. This begins in the form of fatty buildup in the organs, plaque in the arteries, stiffness in the joints and other subtle but telltale symptoms. As the process continues, more serious symptoms arise such as kidney stones, various kinds of cysts, swellings and enlargements, blood clots and much more. Blocked ear passages, clogged sinuses, swollen glands and lymph nodes, pimples, rashes, moles, warts, styes, abscesses, and hemorrhoids are symptoms of excess as well.

Ask people who have been wisely practicing macrobiotic eating for more than five years if they have these symptoms. *You will discover very few who do.* Only those who eat in excess and take concentrated fats, protein, and sugar develop these extreme signs of abnormal elimination. This accumulation of excess energy, if it is continued and not eliminated, will cause many serious health problems. Remember: whatever is consumed must be eliminated. The body's urge is to live. If it is to live it must stay free of accumulation. If it can't rid itself of the accumulation through normal channels, it will find other ways. When the usual channels of elimination are filled and worked to capacity, the body must find additional routes for elimination. These areas, not normally used by the body as areas of elimination, are called upon when the body has become extremely overburdened. Because they provide openings to the surface of the body, here, possibly, excess can be eliminated. The only problem is that these areas, while providing an opening to the surface, don't have active functions to promote elimination, so excess easily gets stuck in these areas as it tries to exit the body. The most often used areas for this overflow of excess and abnormal elimination are as follows:

1. The ears which build up with mucus, fluid and sticky substances.
2. The nasal passages and sinuses which become clogged.
3. The breasts which grow full of fat and accumulations that often turn into cysts and tumors.
4. The prostate gland which gradually becomes hard and swollen due to the accumulating fat and mineral deposits.
5. The uterus, ovaries, and Fallopian tubes which become weakened or blocked by accumulating energy.

The hardening and stiffening that develops in the muscles and joints as a result of this process eventually leads to severe inflexibility throughout the whole body. It may take decades for this to become apparent, but ultimately it does come to those who overconsume, overindulge, and think that somehow they will be the ones who are able to sidestep the laws of nature. Often these people say, "Oh, what difference does it make? Everyone has to get old sometime, everyone gets sick and feeble. Why shouldn't I do as I please?" These are the same individuals who complain constantly when they *are* sick, who need others to push them in wheelchairs, who force their families to sacrifice time because they need pampering while they groan about their aches and pains, and suck vast volumes of energy from whole cadres of doctors, nurses and technicians. Chronic and degenerative illness is the physical result of a life of extreme self-abuse. How well I know. It's not something to feel guilty about. The truth has to be faced before healing can start.

My own case of paranoid schizophrenia is a classic one of illness resulting from gluttony, self-centered living and ignorance of the simple order of life that makes our physical and psychological aspects one unitary movement. What a fool I was to have blamed my problems on others and to have waited for others to solve them. As a consequence, I wasted many years of my young life.

When I was growing up I loved to eat all of the things that any good, hungry American loves. I especially enjoyed candy bars, ice cream and Cokes. I could have as much of them as I wanted, and I wanted plenty. Also, I relished hard, salty, and well-done meats like crispy bacon, fried ham, cheeseburgers, almost-burnt steak, and beef jerky. Anything salty, crispy, and dry made a great snack as far as I was concerned. But mostly it was the sugar I went after. One of my favorite sweet snacks was a mixing bowl full of vanilla ice cream that was covered with half a box of brown sugar. No wonder I went crazy, right? I consumed whole bags of candy bars at one sitting and washed them down with bottles of Coke. My friends loved to spend the day at my house because of the extravagant snacks and lunches I would fix for them. Super supreme pizza? You bet. How about two? No problem. Root-beer floats? Here we come! Chocolate-covered peanuts, syrup, caramel topping, peanut butter cups, butter mints? Oh boy. Brown sugar right from the box? Certainly.

As a result of this kind of eating, my behavior and thinking became neurotic. The sugary stuff had wild effects on my blood sugar, making roller-coaster qualities in my personality. My imagination was uncontrollable. Sometimes I was very cruel, sometimes a sentimenatal slob. Extreme sentimentality can turn into cruelty. My mind was so far out in space that my friends who took drugs loved to be with me because I would conjure up the wildest and most bizarre stories and mental adventures. Through drugs they were trying to get their minds to the place where mine already was!

When I socialized, I became a dozen different personalities. To one friend I'd be a jokester, to another a confidant, to another a scholarly poet, to another I was a cool playboy. Because of the ungrounding effects of the expansive energy of sugar and drugs, I usually didn't know who or what I was. I couldn't concentrate on school studies or anything for very long. I had constantly pervading fears that seemed to jump out of the walls and hallways. Fear is a result of very weak kidneys, and I was always having kidney problems. Once I was hospitalized because of them. I exploded sometimes with great cannonballs of anger. At other times I was overly patient and extremely meek. Sometimes aggressive, I'd bully clerks in stores; at other times I could easily be bullied by others. Passive and lonely, I was game for whatever others wanted me to do. These kinds of ups and downs characterized my life for twenty-two years. I had no idea that I was responsible for this, that through my own mouth every day I was delivering the raw materials for my own mental illness.

The extremely contracting qualities of energy contained in the well-cooked meats, salty chips and hard-boiled eggs contributed greatly to my feelings of tension, frustration and suppressed emotion. They gnawed at my insides so much that I had three duodenal ulcers by the time I was twenty-two. The intense energy in the animal fats and protein could have never been eliminated by one as lazy as I. I hated physical exercise of any kind. I became completely self-centered and obsessed with my own pleasures and needs.

The extremely expanding energy of sugar and most drugs contributed to the decades of passivity that comprised my early life. I cried a lot and felt sorry for myself, and the feeling of not being able to change anything was insufferable. I had dreams and goals, but the lack of calm energy prevented me from charting any direction. There were mostly sad and drifting days.

Since beginning macrobiotics, I have accomplished anything I have dreamed of doing. I discovered that macrobiotics clears the resistance to life's natural movement around us and in us. We are naturally meant to be happy, to accomplish our dreams enjoy the earth, and when one becomes cleaner and clearer through macrobiotic eating, all of life's natural flow moves without interference. If you try it you will see how much more easily a dream can become reality. You have to play with macrobiotics for many years before this becomes really clear. A few years begins to heal the body, but many more years of macrobiotic practice allows healing energy to soak deeply into the mind. Even if you are not seriously mentally ill, macrobiotics can bring about wonderful changes in your mind. Just try it, be patient, and enjoy the days.

Eating a macrobiotic diet that is centered around whole grains and vegetables allows the body to gradually eliminate excess accumulations inside because macrobiotic foods strengthen the organs and offer high-quality nourishment that is free of the loaded fats, sugar, and protein of standard food. Cells and organs are allowed to regain their natural healthy functioning and to do the work they are meant to do. (See the Appendix for an outline of the Standard Macrobiotic Diet.)

You will see as your body becomes healthier, that the various emotional disturbances associated with the imbalance of a particular organ will change, too. Macrobiotics teaches that the following organs and emotions are associated:

Problem Organ	*Associated Emotion*
kidneys/bladder	fear
liver/gall bladder	anger
stomach/spleen-pancreas	anxiety
lungs/large intestine	sorrow
heart/small intestine	joy (excessive laughter)

Please be pateint. The body needs time to heal, and this process of healing can be the greatest adventure of your life.

Two years after I started macrobiotics I came down with a very strange sickness. Everyone around me was certain that I had the flu, but having had the flu many times. This was different. I didn't know it at the time but I was having a classic macrobiotic "discharge." It came in the form of an intense fever that moved in waves from my feet to the top of my head and then back down. I was aware that something unusual was taking place. There was an odd taste in my mouth that was vaguely familiar. I finally identified it as the taste of Thorazine, a psychiatric drug I had taken for many years but gradually discontinued when I started macrobiotics.

The doctors had told me that the Thorazine would be quickly and completely excreted from my body, but here I was still eliminating it many years later. In a few days my fingers broke out with many small, watery blisters which lasted for about one week before disappearing. I was later told that this was a sign of drugs discharging from my body. I was elated. It wasn't until twelve years later, though, that I had the biggest discharge of all.

During a party on a December night in 1984, I began to develop a high temperature which eventually sent me home to bed. I awoke the next morning to the strong odor of medicine all around me. I thought that something must have been spilled on the rug. I wondered what it was. Like the smell of a pharmacy or hospital, it was overpowering. My wife entered the room and told me that the medicinal odor was coming from me! It was there the night before when she returned home and found me asleep. My breath, saliva, hands, feet, and every other part of me oozed this medicinal odor. My eyes throbbed painfully and the area under my lower right ribs ached. The familiar taste of Thorazine was once again in my mouth, and there were tastes of aspirin and other un-identifiable medicines. After about one week these intense symptoms disappeared, and I felt incredibly strong and vital.

There have been no strong symptoms of drug elimination since then. I discovered that drugs and strong medications *do* accumulate in the body, but they can be eliminated through good macrobiotic eating.

My experiences of discharging are not unique. Many who begin macrobiotics experience discharges. This is natural when the body is given the opportunity to cleanse itself of the long-held accumulations of drugs, fats, mucus and chemicals. Most people won't experience the kind of dramatic discharge I had, unless, perhaps, they have consumed strong drugs and medication for years. Most discharging will be more subtle than mine was, usually being taken care of by the normal channels of elimination. But discharge you will, because everything that you have consumed will eventually have to get eliminated.

If you have been taking strong medication or drugs for many years, you must take a wise but steady transition to macrobiotic eating. Most people can't stop long-term dosage of medication overnight, nor is it advisable to do so. I tried to stop six years of strong medication and go on the famous brown rice fast all at the same time. I almost went insane. My weak organs and nervous system could not handle the stress, neither can yours. Please consult with an experienced macrobiotic teacher and the appropriate medical professional in order to adjust the macrobiotic approach to your personal needs.

Without the necessary change to a macrobiotic practice, everything else in this book can be used, but maybe not as successfully. They will just be techniques practiced in a vacuum, a kind of mental meringue. I know, because I have watched hundreds of friends try to get their lives and health together without a concern for daily diet. Yes, a few may have succeeded, but unfortunately the rest are still struggling. *A peaceful and healthy life must be built upon cellular peace.*

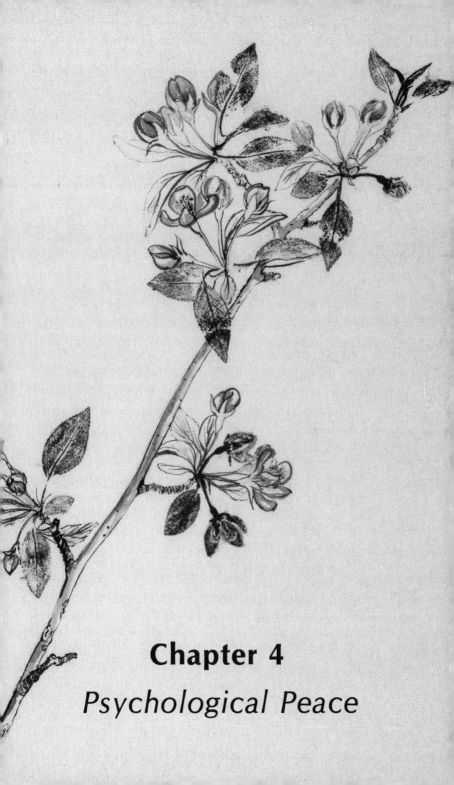

Chapter 4
Psychological Peace

I. ORGANIC PSYCHOLOGY

HEALING THE BODY MUST BE THE FIRST STEP toward healing the mind. If we bypass the body and try to heal the mind directly through meditation, positive thinking, psychoanalysis, etc., our efforts will be constantly undermined. Over the years, I have met with many people who are practicing different techniques of meditation and psychology. Even though they have perfected their techniques after years of study and practice, great numbers of them have complained to me about having an agitated mind and restless, distracted feelings that interfere with their practices.

Often, because of dietary-related tension and inflexibility in the body, they can't sit still or feel physically and mentally relaxed. There are many who proclaim that health is a matter of "mind over body," or who say "take care of the soul, forget about the body." These unfortunate individuals live in their own fragmented world where body and spirit are split apart, rather than whole and inseparable. Such lopsided living and thinking perpetuates imbalance and lack of fulfillment in people's lives.

At the same time there are those involved with physical health, natural nutrition and exercise who become obsessed with food and the body. Macrobiotics has often been criticized for focusing almost exclusively on food as the means of re-covering from any physical and mental problem. Genuine macrobiotics, however, is an all-embracing approach to living, not only eating. Merely eating macrobiotic food products and cooking from macrobiotic recipes hardly makes one fully macrobiotic.

A macrobiotic body must also have a macrobiotic mind. It seems to me that there must be a macrobiotic mind and heart before one can really prepare macrobiotic-quality food and live the genuine macrobiotic way in this world. Our attitude, actions, deeds and relationships are essential aspects of our lives. Much more than our theories, beliefs, ideologies and dreams, our daily living reveals the facts of who we are.

Like cellular peace, macrobiotics views psychological peace as much more than the absence of observable, superficial symptoms of illness. Observable symptoms can, however, tell us much about the physical state that contributes to negative emotional outbursts and psychological manifestations.

For thousands of years, practitioners of traditional Oriental medicine have successfully applied their understanding of the way energy circulates, nourishes, and animates the body. The organs were seen as energy centers which together worked harmoniously to create one united organism. The Chinese first proposed that yin and yang together comprise all phenomena. The ancient practitioners of Oriental medicine developed very precise and sophisticated ways of classifying the organs and their various functions, interactions, and manifestations according to yin and yang energetics. Through careful observation and refinement of these principles over countless generations of practice, they learned the relationship and harmony between body, mind, spirit, and matter. The separating of body from mind was to them unthinkable. The relationship between emotions and organs was too evident and easy to observe in its orderly manifestations.

Today, macrobiotics uses this understanding as a means of gaining practical insight into our own physical and mental health and to discover their interplay. Macrobiotics has developed many of the complex principles of Oriental medicine into practical tools for modern everyday use.

Human behavior is one of the most practical ways of observing and reflecting upon one's state of health. As stated in the previous chapter, the outward symptoms of elimination reveal the inward condition. Emotions, being relatively easy to observe outgoing energy, provide tangible ways for people to begin evaluating their own health. As a simple way of viewing the level of strength or weakness in particular organs, take the following Organ/Emotion Evaluation Test. Take it yourself, and then have someone who knows you very well fill it in according to their past and present observations of you. Often, another's observations of your emotional behavior can be quite helpful.

Organ/Emotion Evaluation

I	II	III	IV	V
Li/GB	Ht/SI	St/Sp–P	Lu/LI	Ki/Bl/RO

On a piece of paper draw five separate columns. Number and letter each one as in the above illustration.

According to how you observe your *overall* behavior and emotional tendencies (not only how you feel right now), mark an X in the respective column for each of the following emotions or types of behavior which applies to you:

I	II	III	IV	V
anger	rigidity	critical	sadness	fear
short temper	easily excited	skeptical	depression	defensiveness
cruelty	nervousness	worry	indecision	hopelessness
violence	agitation	jealous	over-analysis	aloofness
stubbornness	excessive laughter or speech	envy	confusion	coldness
narrow-minded	separation	suspicious	weakness	timid
rigidity	impulsiveness	distrust	low self-esteem	indecisive
rage	hyperactive	self-pity	melancholy	protective
domineering	boisterous	cynical		paranoia
irritable	superficial	over-dependent		threatened
insensitive	erratic	extreme depression		self-protective
over-control		crave constant reassurance		sexual anxiety
tension				

Now take a look at the columns you marked with the most X's. These represent the organs of your body, where, according to the organ/emotion theory, you would need to direct the most healing attention. Of course, the entire physical organism can benefit from an intelligently and appropriately done macro-biotic diet (see the Appendix) along with proper exercise, breathing, sleep, work, and other lifestyle factors. Let's look at each pair of organs and some of the macrobiotic dietary details that are specific to them.

The first column above represents the emotions and be-haviors associated with impaired liver and gallbladder func-tion. The liver and gallbladder are inhibited by the regular consumption of overly contractive foods such as meat, animal fats, salt, eggs, hard cheese, dry and crispy foods like baked bread, crackers and chips. These foods create the hard and tight condition that leads to the emotional manifestations listed in Column I.

In addition, many natural-health enthusiasts suffer because of excessive use of herbal cleansers, spices, fasting, and liver "flush" remedies. By over-stimulating the liver, they are actually making worse the weakness they are trying to heal. Extremely expansive foods such as alcohol, sugar, and drugs will eventually lead to an expanded and hard liver. Regardless of what kind of food one eats, *overeating* is the habit most harmful to the liver. Some overeat macrobiotic food, thinking, perhaps, that because it is organic and natural food it will be good to take more of it. They are unknowingly contributing to the inhibition of their own livers.

In most cases where the liver has become too yang, a shift-ing of the diet to a lighter, good-quality yin direction can be very beneficial. Especially nourishing to an overly yang liver are macrobiotic foods such as whole grains, wheat, barley, leafy green vegetables, lightly cooked vegetables, raw salads, light-strength miso soup, sprouts, *shiitake* mushroom, small amounts of fruit, light-strength pickles, sour foods and natur-ally fermented foods. *With any overly yang condition it is re-commended that the consumption of salt be greatly reduced.* A healthy liver and gall bladder establish patience and endurance.

Column II represents the emotions and behavior associated with the inhibition of the heart and small intestine. Strong, stimulating foods bring excessively activating energies into these organs. Alcohol, citrus drinks, hot and spicy foods, coffee, and drugs have a direct effect on the heart and small intestine. Everyone has experienced the boisterousness that comes to a once quiet crowd after it has been consuming alcohol for an hour or so. Often individuals or cultures who consume regular amounts of hot spices are viewed as "hot-headed," "fiery" and "emotional." In addition, the consumption of animal fat has long been associated with problems relating to the heart and circulatory system.

The condition of the small intestine will greatly determine the body's ability to absorb nutrients. If it has been weakened or overworked by too much eating, ulcers, or surgery, a person often has difficulty maintaining weight. Many such people become quite skinny when changing to macrobiotic eating until they learn how to adjust the diet more appropriately. This is more common among men. In my own case, I lost about thirty pounds after six months of beginning macrobiotics. I felt great compared to how I had been feeling before, but to my friends and relatives I appeared emaciated. After a long history of duodenal ulcers and overeating, my digestive tract was pretty weak. As I gradually strengthened and learned more about proper cooking and food selection techniques, I gained back a normal amount of weight. I didn't worry so much about weight, though, because my mind was getting progressively clearer and more settled the longer I ate macrobiotically. That was much more important to me than the numbers on the bathroom scale.

Macrobiotic foods which are especially nourishing to the heart and small intestine are whole grains, particularly corn, expanded leafy-green vegetables, burdock, *wakame* and *kombu* sea vegetables, and bitter tasting foods. One word of warning: many people take ginseng for a variety of reasons, including sexual problems. Improper use of ginseng, however, can cause heart attack, high blood pressure and stroke. Most Westerners should avoid the use of ginseng because it is too yang. Only an experienced and qualified Oriental herbalist really understands how to properly prescribe ginseng. Fortunately, the ginseng generally used in the United States is not of particularly strong quality. Beware of it nonetheless.

A strong and healthy heart and small intestine will manifest emotionally and behaviorally as gentleness, outgoing, giving, merry or humorous, and a peaceful, cooperative spirit.

The emotions generated by an unhealthy stomach, spleen and pancreas are listed in Column III. Their functions are especially impeded by concentrated and refined forms of sugar, including excess fruit sugar. Yang foods such as eggs, hard, baked flour products, shrimp, chicken, cheese and other animal fats can overstimulate the pancreas leading to hypoglycemia and other pancreatic disorders. Overuse of fatty foods, and pastas and sauces made from refined flour have a gradual but inevitable inhibiting effect on the spleen.

Macrobiotic foods which have been found to be especially nourishing to these organs are yellow millet, squash, onions, cabbage, round vegetables, high-mineral vegetables such as leafy greens and sea vegetables, sweet rice and naturally sweet foods. A lightly cooked quality is much preferred to regular use of salty, dry, baked, and hard quality. When these middle-organs are healthy, understanding, consideration, sympathy, steadfastness and resourcefulness are bound to be present in your behavior and emotional outlook. Daily vigorous exercise which helps the spleen, pancreas, and movement of lymph fluid, should be part of a regular routine depending on one's condition.

The emotions and behavior patterns in Column IV are related to the lungs and large intestine which are adversely affected by excess fluid. Water, coffee, watery fruits, tea, soft and liquidy dairy products taken excessively, lead to the loosening and weakening of the lungs and large intestine. People are usually surprised when they hear that all of this liquid is not good for them because they are constantly encouraged by doctors, nutritionists, and commercials to drink more of everything.

"My kidneys need it," they say. Of course, the body needs liquid, but the excess volumes that people consume are creating vast health problems, especially in the kidneys, lungs, and large intestine. Along with excess liquid, there is the buildup of mucus in the lungs from the regular consumption of dairy products. It is common knowledge that most individuals who have respiratory problems and heavy mucus accumulations throughout the body benefit tremendously from the elimination of dairy products. Besides dairy products, excess consumption of foods that are made from refined flour products like bread, cookies, crackers and pasta, will also contribute to mucus stagnation in the lungs and large intestine.

Good chewing is one of the best investments you can make in the health of your large intestine. People who chew really well (50 times or more per mouthful) cut in half the time necessary to realize benefits from macrobiotic eating. *There is nothing more beneficial to overall health than good chewing.* Macrobiotics recommends brown rice, watercress, cauliflower, lotus root, ginger, *daikon*, kale, scallions and other naturally pungent foods for the lungs and large intestine. Exercises which involve breath control are highly recommended for everyone, especially people who have a tendency for depression, and *hara* (abdominal) massage throughout the entire abdominal area has been found very helpful for the large intestine. Positiveness, practicality, unity, and security permeate one whose lungs and large intestine become strong and healthy.

Column V represents emotions and behavior related to unhealthy kidneys, bladder and reproductive organs. People who have strong kidneys and bladders are confident, adventurous, curious and courageous. However, the kidneys are weakened by the regular consumption of cold foods and drinks such as iced beverages, ice cream, foods eaten directly from the refrigerator, cold sodas, and sugary drinks. Regular use of tropical fruit drinks, nightshade vegetables such as potato and tomato, spinach, and other extremely yin vegetables contribute to the diminishing of healthy kidney function. Excess fluids are also a stress to the kidneys. Very clearly, when the kidneys become weak, our willpower and determination are impaired, and we are filled with a variety of fears.

Salt can be a help or hindrance depending upon what kind of kidney vitality a person has. Study of macrobiotic books, or the advice of an experienced macrobiotic teacher can help you to better understand the most appropriate way to use salt for good health.

Macrobiotic foods which generally benefit weak kidneys are whole grains, especially buckwheat, *azuki* and other beans, and sea vegetables. It can't be stressed enough, though, that for the kidneys, learning the most appropriate use of salt is very important. Barefoot walking has been found to be excellent for strengthening weak kidneys as is any kind of barefoot garden work.

I have presented some of the most basic information about the organs and their relationship to certain emotions according to traditional macrobiotic theory. It can take awhile before you becomes personally sensitive to this organ/emotion relationship, but if you study it more and observe yourself and others, you will gradually begin to perceive it. Experience will be your best teacher, and eventually you will clearly see how the way you eat affects particular organs and emotions. For an in-depth presentation of the way energy, food, organs, emotions and behavior are connected, please read *Macrobiotics and Human Behavior* by William Tara.

II. THE OTHER SIDE OF THE COIN

Through my own experience, I have discovered two important and complementary approaches to psychological peace. The first I have already discussed. It involves the following:

1. Effort (dietary changes, exercise, self-education, reorganizing one's schedule, socializing, etc.)
2. Time
3. Patience.

This is the yang, physical side of establishing psychological peace. It takes determination and willpower. The body requires time to really heal as nature intended it to, and macrobiotic dietary changes will eventually bring about deep emotional healing. Most of this emotional healing will be subtle, taking place over a long period of time. Only when you look back after some years of macrobiotic practice will it be startlingly apparent. Sometimes, dramatic emotional changes will be quickly evident after a wise and consistent beginning practice of macrobiotics. However, the majority of psychological healing takes place over a period of about seven to eight years. While long-term physical and emotional healing is taking place, though, there are still the daily emotional realities to deal with. I continued to experience serious mental and emotional problems during my first years of macrobiotic practice, but it was clear that they were diminishing in intensity as my ability to cope with them was growing stronger.

The other side to psychological peace is the yin, spiritual counterpart to the physical, yang approach. It is characterized by the following:

1. No effort to change psychologically, no self-suppression
2. Sensitive awareness and self-reflection
3. Inward blossoming.

Emotional patterns and long-time modes of behavior and thinking don't change overnight. In fact, malignant tumors have been known to dissolve more quickly through macrobiotic healing than deeply held emotional and psychological stagnation.

If you observe your feelings, thinking, and emotions you will discover that a tremendous amount of energy is wasted in

rying to change, deny, suppress or escape from what you are
ictually feeling. Feelings and emotions are not in and of them-
elves so painful and difficult; what does cause great pain,
hough, is the battle we make to deny, change, condemn and
idge ourselves for the feelings and emotions we experience.

For example, at the very moment we feel anger, there is
he complete immersion in the feeling. It is neither good nor
ad, right nor wrong. It is simply there, mildly or with great
orce. Within a few seconds of feeling anger, though, we begin
o put ourselves through a whole battery of thoughts. We say,
'I shouldn't have been angry," or "I must try harder to be
nderstanding and patient." We try to rationalize the anger,
orget about it, push it away, or feel guilty. All of this struggle
o change what one is feeling creates great tension, clutter, and
latter in the mind. Feelings and emotions are kept smoldering
nside the mind because they are not allowed to fully blossom
nd naturally wither away. Great honesty must be present in
ou if you are going to be able to see yourself exactly as you
re throughout the day.

The most important first step for arriving at the under-
tanding that all psychological effort to change oneself actually
revents change from occurring, is to begin watching how
nuch you struggle to change, deny, avoid and dismiss what
ou are doing and feeling. You will be very surprised to
iscover that you are struggling against yourself. Just relax
nd watch yourself in all of your relationships to people,
vents and things. The only way to end this constant inner
attling is to become intensely aware of it. Don't try to stop
truggling. Don't say to yourself, "I must not struggle in
rder to be healthy." Simply observe your own attempts to
eny what you are actually feeling and experiencing. When
ou so observe yourself, you will begin to see that your mind
tarts to relax, and you can feel at ease with the facts of
ourself.

A seed, if it is to naturally change into a flower, must be
iven the right soil, nutrients, and space in which to sprout,
row, blossom, and wither away. It is natural for a seed to do

this. If it is inhibited or crowded it can't fulfill its life cycle, and it remains incomplete. It is the same with feelings and emotions. If they are not allowed to "bloom," they remain hidden and stuck inside, creating all kinds of problems.

A feeling or emotion will reveal itself to you and teach you all of its details and nuances if you will just leave it alone. As soon as you try to change it, act upon it, or suppress it, you have clipped it back. Its energy will go deep inside you, and you will not have directly contacted it, seen its colors as it unfolds, and watched it naturally, effortlessly wither away.

Space is very important to a healthy mind. My first macrobiotic cooking teacher advised me to "be empty" if I wanted to cook really delicious macrobiotic food. When asked how he performed his daily activities with such ease and good humor, Michio Kushi responded, "Be empty." Krishnamurti challenged us to "empty the mind of its content" if we are to live in wholeness. Every great teacher has said in one way or another that we must become empty if we are to really discover how to play and be happy on this earth.

My own experience has shown that they are absolutely right. As the body becomes "empty" of excess, it becomes light, flexible and more youthful. Proper macrobiotic eating does bring this sense of positive and vibrant physical emptiness. Fasting has been one of the major healing tools of natural medicine for thousands of years. Carefully done, it can have positive effects on the body and mind. Psychological emptiness can also bring equally healthy changes to the mind.

Unlike the physical emptiness brought to the body through fasting, psychological emptiness requires no effort or regimen, only honesty, awareness, and openness. Excess in the mind becomes heavier and more entrenched when any effort to get rid of it or avoid it is made. The mind can only change and become empty when it is given space, and when one relaxes and watches oneself actively in daily life. We are always trying to change who we are rather than actually observing and contacting the truth of who we are. Only when you make actual contact with what you are doing, thinking, feeling, relating and behaving can it change. The denial of one's actual truth prevents any real psychological change from taking place.

Relax. Learn about yourself day to day. Forget about who you were yesterday or what you plan to be tomorrow. Find out about yourself right now. If you closely observe, you will see that all psychological pain comes from dwelling on what has happened or what you imagine will happen tomorrow. What is going on inside of you right now is who you are. Just observe your own self, free of the desire to change yourself, judge yourself, or act upon what you observe. You will find that an amazing freedom to be exactly who you are now comes into being. The following chapter, *Sound, Silence, and Solitude* and the chapter on *Ki-Yō*, further explores the need for an empty and quiet mind if there is to be true psychological peace.

Chapter 5
Sound, Silence, And Solitude

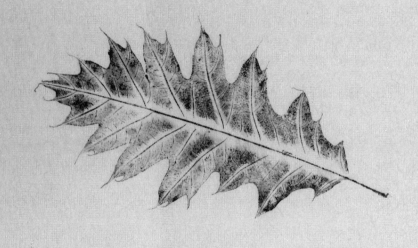

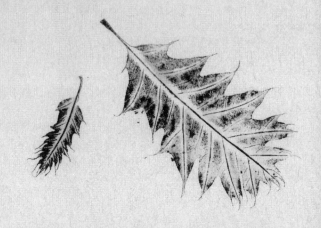

I HAVE FOUND THREE PRECIOUS GEMS. They have many facets, and I have benefited from them for years. I want to give them to you, but that would be impossible. You have to find them for yourself, and if you are lucky enough to come upon them, you will know what I mean when I write that *sound*, *silence*, and *solitude* are great beauties.

Today, noise is everywhere around us and in us. We create noise to drive away our mental chattering, to fill the lonely intervals of the day, and drown the sorrows and memories that bob on the surface of the brain. There is a constant seeking of outside noise in hopes that the inner noise of one's own pain, discontent, and daily fritterings will be crowded from consciousness. The nagging fear of death is covered by all of our noises. It can't be completely drowned out, though. It is there in the background of consciousness like the tick of a clock in a quiet, dark room.

There is the noise of the TV, radio, stereo, movies, a library with its ideas, bars, parties, conventions, and the list could go on endlessly. There is the noise of politicians and priests, promises, authorities and experts, and there is that ancient noise of weapons and hatred roaring down through the generations of war. It is a noise we seem to love very much as we're always turning up its volume.

I hoped, like most people, that all of this noise would make life easier and more gratifying. It gave me the illusion of being awake, really alive. I have discovered, though, that all of this stimulating noise actually made me dull. It's true, the greater the stimulation the greater the dullness that follows. Dull people are addicted to stimulation. In the midst of the wildest and most stimulating and glamorous situations you will find the most lackluster human beings. Next time take a look. Maybe you are one of them without realizing it.

The sound of life is quite different than noise. Only through real listening can you hear it. Mostly, when we say we are listening, it is a very superficial and distracted kind of *hearing* that is going on, not true listening. We hear what is important to us personally and block out everything else. We hear with the background of our prejudices, and we react with conditioned responses. When we hear someone speaking, we don't pay attention, so obsessed are we with our own ideas and upcoming responses. The cacophany of the self, that tremendous racket of our own thoughts and desires, prevents real listening.

Just like everyone else, I have tried to dodge that voice inside which comes in those lonely moments between noises and asks:"What are you doing with your life? Are you wasting the short years? Are you happy? Do you enjoy your days?" We don't like to hear that voice, so we shake it off and return to a life lost in the loud noises.

Listening from nowhere is the only possible way to really hear the sound of life. Listening from nowhere means listening to everything for the first time. Don't listen *from* yourself, but listen *to* yourself. Listen to your judgments and condemnations. Listen to your jealousy, envy, and greed. Listen to them as they come along. Don't do anything to them, just listen to their song. Listen to your wanting to change everything. Listen to your reactions, responses, thoughts and opinions. Hear their tone and volume. Listen to your gossip and small talk. For the first time, listen to your desire to possess someone, have power over someone, own something. Don't try to chase after what you hear, it would be like trying to chase the sound of a breeze through the trees. Let the sounds of oneself arise and subside like music. When you listen with such awareness, you will see that what you hear becomes completely transformed.

One of the simplest ways to learn about the beauty of listening is to begin with nature. Take a walk and listen to everything around you. Hear the birds and other animals, the voices of children, the movement of the leaves, and the bark of dogs or the call of crickets. The movement of life is all around you, can you hear it? Don't concentrate on any particular sound, but listen to the ebb and flow of the far away and the close. Don't try to identify sounds, just open your senses to the sound of nature. Awaken to the chirps, the crunches, hops and slitherings. The flutters and flurries are there, too, and they are wonderful when you listen as though you never heard them before. There is the sound of the still deer alone in an open field and an unmoving frog on the edge of a pond. There is the sound of the sun as it rises, and the totally different sound of its setting. The seasons as they cycle have sound. Can you hear it? It is not imagined or projected. It is there to delight in when you listen from nowhere.

Through listening to nature without any motive or direction, sensitivity arises to the psychological noise of one's own mind. Without listening to nature, it is probably impossible to hear the self. If you want, you can listen to yourself with the same freshness that lets you hear the bird pecking at the branch or the midnight rain. Listen without intention or concentration to hear what you say and think. Can you hear the voices of long ago telling you who you are, the meaning of life, what you should do and get? Listen to your chatter about what you should do next, say next, and think next. Listen to the whole song of yourself throughout the day. Follow the melody as it moves along.

When I began to listen in this way, I could hear the beat of my own drum. I heard and continue to hear the sound of the truth of my own life. Nobody can hear that sound for me. Nobody can hear your sound for you. You have to listen for yourself. It is such a careful listening, so attentive, like listening for the sounds of survivors in the rubble of a collapsed building. If you so listen, your own rescue has begun.

Silence: Because we have collected so much noise around us and in us, is it possible to have a silent mind? It seems to me that a silent mind is essential to a healthy life. There is the silence of caves and the silence one hears between songs when a record album is playing. Silence lingers in the late night air among the houses, and it settles on the snowy lawns and streets before being tramped by boots. There are such soothing and calming silences in nature if you are sensitive to their presence.

Some experts say we'd go insane if there were always silence, and they've done experiments in which people were blindfolded and had their ears plugged to see what the effects of total silence would be. There are people who pay to be put into floatation tanks in order to find silence, relaxation, and to escape from the demands and responsibilities of daily life. Others seek the refuge of mountains and churches where they hope to find a moment of silence. It is possible to seal out all external noises and create a silent corner away from the loud world, but would that bring about the kind of silence that is the essence of a truly quiet mind?

We human beings have been searching for a silent mind for thousands of years. The spiritual paths, religions, and techniques of psychology pronounce that their way is the one that will bring you your long-awaited still and silent mind. After practicing all of these methods are we silent, or have we only suppressed the noise for awhile until we go out into the world again?

The ritual and repetition of memorized prayers do suppress one's mental noise for the time being. Meditation routines and self-improvement techniques do induce a kind of mechanical quiet. Drugs will briefly submerge the noises of the mind. Such mufflings of the mind's racket are very attractive to today's crowd of confused, over-stimulated, and pleasure-seeking people. Is silence, though, merely the temporary quieting of noises? Does forced quietness bring true silence to the mind?

Silence cannot be induced. Effort can never produce inward silence. The effort to achieve silence is itself a noise in the mind. There is the effort to be holy, the effort to be spiritual, the effort to be peaceful, the effort to achieve a pleasing meditative experience, and the effort to stick out of the crowd. All of these efforts make noise in the mind. There is the noise of ambition, and all of the noises that arise through the effort to become a good person.

I have sought silence and peace ever since I was a boy. I would lie in my room and cry for some kind of quietness to come to my mind. I could hardly bear the noise of my thoughts and frustrations, and I longed, ached, for just one silent night. I hounded others and tried to extract peace and serenity from those I admired. At various times I thought that by closing myself off from others, silence would somehow magically appear. I slept away entire days, thinking that such numbness would silence my mind. Through chasing power, prestige, money, education, and position, I imagined that I could achieve peace of mind. Peace of mind and silence never showed up, only the nightmare of noises.

I have discovered that the first step toward a silent mind is to watch the demand and effort to find silence. All effort will push the peace of silence away from your mind not bring it closer. What is important is not hunting down silence, but the attention to that which prevents silence. Relax. Stop fighting for peace of mind. Take a look at your own inner war.

We have all been taught that we have to win the battle inside ourselves, but if we stop and look at it, this struggle to win and to overcome only creates its own battle and more struggling. Why not just observe the battle, learn about it, and let it end? This may come as a shock, because we've been taught to strive to become better and better. Don't strive, unless you want more struggle. Often, when I discuss this, many people think I'm suggesting that they just sit around and do nothing with their lives. This couldn't be farther from the truth. When seeking, struggling to achieve, hoping to be recognized, fighting to find peace, and struggling for more possessions comes to an end, there is tremendous energy for living a creative life. Struggling, and seeking personal position, fame, or power *is* doing nothing with your life, and this is the way many of us are living. Look at your own life.

The peace of silence never enters through the door of effort, but it is there when the demands to be somebody are dropped. It is there when egoistic ambition stops. It comes in the door when the seeking for power goes out. It blossoms when the chattering mind is left alone, not suppressed or whipped into submission. No one and nothing can give you that silence. A silence that is given or received from something eventually brings its own noise. True silence is the doorway through which the Infinite enters.

Solitude: Solitude and health go hand in hand. A balanced mind and body require solitude. Without them we become physically and mentally crowded, and when we become crowded we eventually explode.

Look at the crowded cities with people living practically on top of each other. See your own crowded mind so full of ideas, opinions, expectations, memories, and demands for more things. Observe the crowding of the brain with the images from TV, movies, and magazines. Even during sleep the pent-up feelings, images, and intimations, seep out in dreams and nightmares.

Why have we crowded ourselves so? Is it in hopes of squeezing out our loneliness? Through overworking, alcohol, drugs, sex, do we hope to hide from that fact of deep loneliness? Look at your relationships. Are they relationships of love or merely ways of filling up the otherwise lonely hours? The entertainment industry caters to our desire to escape loneliness. Amusement parks, sports arenas, concert halls, and nightclubs are packed on account of it. Take a look at your own activities and see for yourself. Most people are frightened of their own loneliness. Many people panic when the weekend approaches and they've nothing planned to do or no one scheduled to be with.

Loneliness has to be faced or it will never disappear from your life. The only way I have ever been able to resolve a problem is by heading straight into it. Every human being knows this ache of loneliness. Is it possible to remain with it long enough to dissolve it, and not run from it? Can you be with it without saying to yourself, "This is loneliness" or "I shouldn't be lonely"? Can you just *be* the loneliness as it arises in you? Out of curiosity try it sometime and see what happens.

Loneliness cannot be put off forever. Why wait for loneliness to sneak up on you by surprise or through the shock of losing a loved one or close friendship? Bring it out now since it is right there smoldering inside you. By looking at it, getting to know it, understanding it, you transform it. So, go ahead, feel your loneliness. Its ending comes when you begin to be aware of it without wishing it away. When something that has been suppressed is allowed to be free, to live, it can naturally grow wither and die. Let this happen with loneliness and you will see that instead of staying half alive and smoldering inside of you, it comes out, blossoms forth, and dies.

Look at the way you use others to cover up your own loneliness. Look at how you imitate others. Be aware of your own urge to conform, and the reaction to conformity usually creates its own conformity. The real pain of loneliness is created by the effort to escape from it. Look and see for yourself.

Being alone is completely different from loneliness. Alone means not being psychologically tethered to anyone or anything. Alone is breaking through one's attachments to belief, nationality, and other forms of group identification. Alone means having no psychological or spiritual authority. Alone means being free to learn who you are moment to moment rather than a slave to memories, psychological experts, and theories about yourself. Alone is to live with intense honesty in one's heart. Alone is to be free of the pressure to achieve personal success and power. Living without expectation is to be vitally alone. Don't mistake the state of being alone as the same as cutting oneself off from friends and other people. A person in a state of withdrawal is not alone, because being alone means being at the center of life, completely free to feel its freshness and verve. Alone is to touch moments that have never been before.

When you are alone, your relationship to everything changes. From others you want nothing, things are enjoyed but not possessed, what you do is what you love to do.

Solitude is the mother of aloneness. Sadly, most people seem to have no time for genuine solitude. Often it is perceived as a luxury or a waste of time. But each human being needs solitude. Like dry ground calling to water, the crowded body and mind wait for solitude.

Ever since I was a boy, the call for solitude has come whenever I felt the need for healing myself. During walks through country fields or down my own street, or driving in a car, solitude has offered the opportunity to look, hear, and feel what is going on inside my mind and outside in the world. I could not have found the kind of life I have without solitude to deepen my understanding and awareness. Solitude slows the mind and gives one the chance to see the whirls of thought and images. Without solitude we become distracted, agitated, and frustrated participants in the confusing pressures of daily life. With solitude the psychological pressures are ended.

Solitude is the birthplace of deep sensitivity to life. I hope you have it daily. Go for walks. Go to your room. Look at yourself in solitude. Soon you will discover that solitude permeates your whole day. It will be there even in the midst of the screeching cities and crowds. You will discover something which you never dreamed of.

Chapter 6

Introducing Ki-Yō: Activities For Psychological Purification

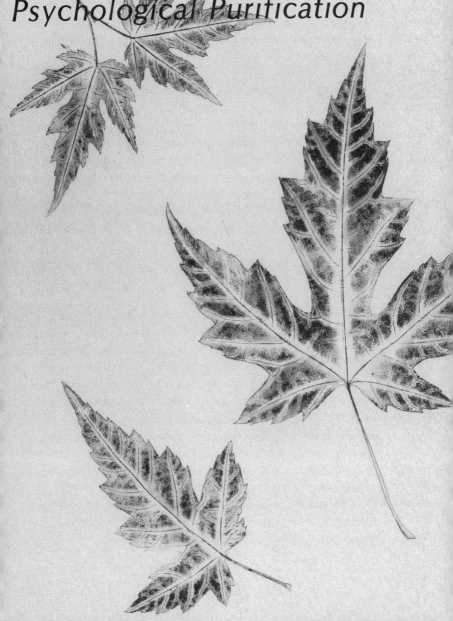

I AM INTRODUCING THE KI-YŌ (key-yoh) APPROACH to psychological purification in order to share with others the most helpful non-dietary factors I have discovered for creating a healthy mind and personal peace. It goes hand in hand with other macrobiotic practices.

These activities are useful for relaxing the mind, opening it, and emptying the mental stagnation that leads to depression, emotional turmoil, confusion, isolation, and the deep unhappiness of self-centered living.

Rather than a series of rigid rules, or dictates to force oneself into a routine of practice, Ki-Yō is an approach consisting of various activities and proposals for self-reflection and self-investigation. It provides possibilities for moving beyond the barriers of egotistic separation and into deeper relationship with humanity, nature, and the entire universe. Ki-Yō is an aid for living macrobiotically, which really means living with sensitivity to and in communion with all of life. There is nothing secretive or mysterious about it, nor is it a "new religion." It is common-sense living.

If you force yourself to practice the Ki-Yō activities, you will find their benefits elusive. Don't push Ki-Yō into your life. If you relax in your approach, you will see that it flows by itself.

No doubt about it, physical activity has been proven beneficial to physical and psychological health. I highly recommend regular physical activity that is appropriate for one's condition and capacity. There are many teachers and services available to help a person discover which kind of physical activity is best suited to his or her needs. Please consult with them. I prefer macrobiotic-style exercises which address the orderly flow of energy within the body, rather than exercise that merely tones muscles or builds superficial strength. There are many books on such holistic exercise, and most macrobiotic centers regularly offer classes in these methods.

This chapter addresses activity and exercise of a different nature. Where maintaining most programs often takes great force and willpower, Ki-Yō is just the opposite—no force, no struggle, and no resistance. It has evolved after many years of my searching for and experimenting with numerous approaches to mental and emotional stability. Ki-Yō is practical and subtle, and its benefits are endless when it is done without the sense of mechanical routine, ritual, or dread with which many people approach exercise programs or meditation and self-improvement techniques.

Since this is a basic introduction, I have selected some of the most essential aspects for discussion here. A future volume must be written in order to give a complete and detailed presentation of all aspects of Ki-Yō.

The main thrust of these activities is the dissolving of that quality of hardness which pervades all levels of our lives, creates blockage of spiritual energy, and leads to the delusion of separation from humanity, nature, and the cosmos. Many of us are riddled with this physical and spiritual hardness and insensitivity. The effects of the modern diet centered around animal protein, fat, sugar, and chemicalized food ultimately result in a body that is increasingly inflexible, insensitive, and lacking in adaptability. This is displayed dramatically in conditions such as arthritis, hardening of the arteries, and a general trend toward stiffening of the body in the young as well as the elderly.

A sensitive body quickly responds to the internal presence of substances which are inappropriate, excessive, or potentially damaging. The fact that millions of people can ingest the large quantities of poor-quality food and dangerous, artificial substances in the modern everyday diet without noticing their immediate effects on the body is an ominous signal of the degree of physical insensitivity present in today's human population.

Can we be truly sensitive to anything beyond ourselves when we are not even sensitive to our own bodies? No wonder there is such insensitivity to the land, the beauty of the trees, cleanliness of our waters, clean air, and each other!

A sensitive body is responsive, not only to what is eaten, but also keenly in touch with what is around it—sound, nature, atmospheric conditions, sights, people, animals, thoughts, moods, and so on. Active and fully alive senses are the result of a highly sensitive and intelligent body.

Physical hardness and diminishing sensitivity is paralleled in the mind where there is a pervading presence of mental tightness, buried fear, and a closing in of one's energy and consciousness into a narrow concrete corral of limited capacity. Physical and mental hardness create a resistance to change and separate us from each other. This hardness and narrowness blocks the smooth flow of the natural life force, resulting in physical inflexibility and modern psychological delusions such as the separate sense of self, separate countries, separate ideologies, separate religions, and the like.

The hardening and narrowing of one's energy produces an obsessive focus on oneself. Wherever we look, there is this pressure and encouragement towards a narrower and narrower concentration of energy which results in the delusion of a separate, ossified, and permanent self.

Many modern psychological techniques emphasize the development of a strong positive sense of self in order to overcome mental and emotional problems. I disagree with this approach. It only adds more support to the delusion of a separate self seeking its own permanent position, personal power, and recognition among the millions of other fragmented selves. Any approach that strengthens the idea of self separate from the rest of humanity inevitably contributes more chaos, mental illness, and subtle violence to that which it is hoping to resolve. This development of and emphasis on the separate self is the greatest spiritual obstacle to the healthy absorption of energies passing through us from Infinity. This delusion of separateness and personal superiority is the primary mental illness that has been spreading through modern people for the last several hundred years.

Today's educational system encourages and promotes an individualism that is based on developing a competitive, comparative, and separative sense of self, while at the same time it struggles to instill an ethic of cooperation and social consciousness. In other words, "love your neighbors," and at the same time do all you can to be better than them, ahead of them, and have as much or more as they do. Strange, isn't it?

Support and reward for this egocentric mentality is received not only in the educational system, but at home, in the church (*my* salvation, *my* place next to God, *my* beliefs, etc.) on TV, commercials and advertisements. I am reminded of the words of a George Harrison song: "All through the day, I, me, mine, I, me, mine!"

This hard and narrow mentality is so tight (yang) that its greedy appetite for further support and identity is voracious. This creates further delusion of separateness such as: *my* nation, *my* religion, *my* possessions, *my* race, *my* family."

It is this self-centered and fragmented mentality that tries to bring about world peace, ecumenism, and all the other futilities that are going on. This is the mentality that goes out into the day-to-day world hoping to have deep relationships or successful marriages. This is the mentality that thinks it can bring a new age to the consciousness of man!

This hardness causes the mind to snap shut when it encounters new ideas and differences in others, and it keeps people separate and longing for love. Such an incredible tightness and focus on oneself produces deep tension of rigid expectations and the steady conflict between one's immobile self-image and the image of what one would like to be, or thinks he or she should be. Most aren't even aware of this hardness and mental stagnation because it is so deeply conditioned in the mind. It can be dissolved, though, and you will be amazed at what happens in your life as it does.

The Ki-Yō activities to be introduced in this chapter are: the Dissolving of Images, Freedom to Learn, Appreciation, and Aware Care.

Dissolving of Images/Freedom to Learn: Each of us has acquired a powerful self-image, either positive or negative, which is accepted as "me." Concentrated and hard, this self-image is with us at all times. It is who you *think* you are.

From this self-image one takes a rigid stand against the outside world. It is interesting to take a brief self-image inventory. Reflect for a moment, then write up to ten characteristics that best describe you as you think of yourself.

There is an enormous amount of past conditioning contributing to this self-image—how your parents raised you, how you have been treated by your peers, society's attitude (i.e. if you conform or don't conform to society's norms), education, religion, tradition, culture, and your own attitude about yourself.

Over the years, the self-image has been programmed into each person's consciousness by these factors in the same way that a computer is programmed. This knowledge is stored in memory and retrieved as thought, or brought out in one's conditioned reactions and pre-programmed responses to experiences, people, and situations. Because of this automatic self-image based on knowledge and memory, we go about the day responding and reacting mechanically to all that is around us. Our conditioned reactions and programmed thinking crank from our consciousness like a computer print-out:

"I can't do anything right . . . click . . . I'm a helpless person . . . click . . . ," or "I'm important . . . I have money . . . I'm powerful . . . zip . . . click . . . Take care of me first . . . ," "I'm macrobiotic," and I look down on the poor unfortunate, non-American, non-Christian, non-macrobiotic and misinformed people.

Conditioned responses repeat themselves daily. *Are you a computer, robot, or a free human being?* This embedded self-image and stagnant consciousness prevent us from being totally alive, fully conscious, and dynamic. You can't learn about yourself and flow freely with living changes if you are trapped in the dead concept known as "me."

If you look closely and sensitively, you will see that your self-image is merely a conglomeration of festering memories, knowledge, and thoughts. Your mind is packed with all of them, and you accept this mechanically recorded program, this racket of rote responses, as the truth of who you are.

Who you imagine yourself to be and who you actually are could be totally different. How can we come into direct contact and awareness of these stifling images and other mental pre-programming? I suggest the following approach:

1. Spend a day as you go about your regular activities being aware of your self-image as it reveals itself in your thoughts, actions, motives, and behavior.

2. It can be very helpful to keep track of these observations by having a pocket-size notebook where you can jot down the observations when you have the opportunity. Or, at the end of the day, enter your thoughts as a kind of diary of what you observed about your self-image during the day.

3. Record the many different ways your self-image showed itself: "I'm an American, a Jew, a Christian; I'm neglected, I'm an expert, I'm always lazy, I'm not smart, I can't."

4. Also watch how much of what you do is done because you *think* you have to do it in order to conform to what you have been *told*, *educated*, or *indoctrinated* to do. Is what you do in the course of a day the clear response of your own free perception and clear consciousness? How much is merely computer-like response to mental pre-programming? Are you living freely, or are you on automatic pilot? People who are programmed and running on automatic pilot are heading straight into the mountain-side of personal and social conflict.

5. Spend one day fasting psychologically. That is, watch the self-image program you observed the previous day. When you see the same behavior and thoughts arising in yourself today, be aware of them. Don't suppress them and don't feed them energy. Watch them coming forth and let them show themselves. For example, if you observed yourself being critical yesterday, and you also generally consider yourself a chronically critical person, yet you realize clearly,

all the dangers of destructive criticism, then watch
intensely your criticism today. Continue to watch the
urge to criticize or gossip when it arises, but in seeing
it intensely, you transform it.

Don't feel guilty if you keep on criticizing or gossiping,
just be completely aware of it. When you become conscious
of the workings of your own mind, *the awareness itself* opens
and empties it. Just be patient. Play with it.

As you begin to actually see your self-image and the images
you have of others, you will naturally become aware of the
multitude of ways in which you have corralled yourself into
one small and limited corner. We are frustrated, suppressed,
and spiritually frozen by such limitations. The human heart is
a wild and beautiful fire that must be allowed to burn bright
and free.

Take a different issue each day and watch to see if the rigid
images of yourself and others emerge and create stagnation.
Make a list of various aspects of daily life and watch a different
one closely each day. The following list can be used as a guide:

1. Relationships
2. View of men
3. Attitude towards women
4. Attachment to beliefs
5. Attitude towards strangers versus attitude towards
   friends
6. Attitude towards next-door neighbors and neighbors
   thousands of miles away
7. Attitude towards nature and the environment
8. People you dislike
9. Prejudices
10. Religious images

In simple, everyday situations, watch how your own embedded self-image, and images you have of others color all
that you do. For example, watch when you are driving. Do

you actively participate in the whole situation that you are in, or do you make it a "me against the world" approach? Is the only issue of importance the one of *your* destination? Are you aware of the needs and safety of the other drivers? Is everyone in *your* way?

When you exit a building, do you let the door slam in the face of the person following you? Are you even aware, in simple day-to-day situations, that there are other human beings in the world besides yourself? Responsibility means the ability to properly respond. Are *you* responsible? Do *you* respond?

When you see scenes of war and suffering on television is it someone else's problem or fault? Are you responsible for the whole or are you a hermetically sealed self in an isolated orbit? Complicated analysis is not necessary. Simply look and see for yourself.

Observe when you approach an acquaintance with whom you've had some previous conflict. Feel your stomach tighten and your pulse rate quicken as your images of the past conflict and the present encounter arise to cloud your present relationship with that person. Such automatic responses prevent you from changing and approaching the relationship fresh and clean as it exists now. As the old images arise, let go of them by being intensely and non-judgmentally aware of their presence. Such effortless awareness prevents their inhibiting energy from gaining momentum.

When we really see the ever-present and enslaving nature of our rigid images, we eliminate their burden from our minds. The mind begins to relax, open, and have space and sensitivity. Your true nature is free to manifest itself moment to moment.

As I began to discover the nature of my self-image, I realized just how much tension and anger I was harboring as a result of being in this prison. I thought, as many others have, that I was unworthy, unloveable, and useless. I was trapped within the walls of my own "I can'ts," "I won'ts," and "I shouldn'ts."

The "me" who I imagined myself to be was the programmed self-image in my consciousness. Each person has a pro-grammed self-image. Some are negative, others positive. Many of today's self-improvement programs recommend replacing one's negative self-image with a positive one through a variety of methods and exercises. I completely disagree with this approach, because we are not machines to be programmed— even positively. We are natural, alive, and changing beings whose hearts must have freedom and fluid comprehension of life. Any kind of programming of the human mind crystalizes it and severely limits its scope and capacity for living fully.

Psychologically, when I say, "I know who I am," and I cut from knowledge a frozen image of myself, I am blocking the freedom of living and learning from *right now*. If you once discover what it means to live with a wide open mind, you cannot live with a fixed self-image or images of others.

If I say to myself, "It's the same old me," I've stopped learning about myself and there is no chance for change. But if I watch, listen, and learn from my thoughts, actions, and behaviors as they occur, I am free to move with the changing reality. Through this approach to learning about oneself comes the release into life's true and fluid nature.

Like a child who is sparked with attention and curiosity, you can watch and learn about yourself, never holding onto what you learn, so that learning is continuous movement, incapable of accumulating into a rigid self-image or other stagnant energy in the mind.

The great majority of us think, "I would be lost without my self-image. It is all I know or have. I'd go crazy without it!" Or, "If I don't have a religious, racial, or national identity I'd be nobody, a nothing." Don't feel ashamed or guilty if you have a similar response. Just be *aware* of your responses and see them for what they are. One begins to discover the stranglehold on consciousness that one's conditioned ideas, identities, and prejudices have.

Macrobiotics is not only learning about the necessity of discharging accumulated chemicals, cysts, toxins, mucus, and fat from the body, but also seeing the importance of discharging the accumulated, pre-programmed and conditioned mentali

from the mind—the psychological cysts and mental mucus that
clog the consciousness. In the same way that we discover
through macrobiotics which food energy and nourishment is
appropriate to a fully functioning physical organism, we should
be actively aware of the psychological factors which produce
a healthy, free, and unlimited mind and of those which inhibit
it.

Many of us hop from one belief system to another, thinking
that we are free and creative because we have changed our
mode of thinking. Isn't what we have done, though, a mere
settling into another mode of thinking and living until we
become bored and exchange it for another habit of belief?
Apparently for some, macrobiotics also becomes another in
a long, drawn out series of hops from one belief to another,
blindly accepted for awhile and then tossed aside.

Such flip-flopping of belief systems is not freedom at all.
Free living means not being bound to any belief system, but
living with tremendous intensity, questioning, doubting,
looking, and listening to see and hear the truth as it moves.
Any belief system creates a solidified stand that is inflexible,
divisive, and incapable of receiving that which is always new—
life itself. Free living is being of the moving whole, not
stagnating in fragments. This is *one* earth, *one* air, *one* water,
and *one* family. It is not *American* earth, *Jewish* air, or *Catholic*
water; not *my* family. This fragmented, self-centered, and
essentially mentally ill frame of mind is destroying our earth,
skies, water, and our brothers and sisters. Why do we hang
onto it so ferociously? Why do we cling to our identity with
a religion, a country, a race, or a culture? Can we not see
that it is going to destroy the world if such a mentality
continues? Almost everyone continues to pass along the
centuries-old myth that the fragments will soon get together
and create a unified and peaceful world. This kind of thinking
is total nonsense. The fragmentary, self-centered mind can't
create wholeness, health, or one peaceful world. Is our self-
centeredness so powerful, so deceptive and hypnotizing that we

are unable to see it? As long as each one is seeking his or her own separate pleasure, power, and recognition, the world will be as it is now. This hard, self-centered mentality is the source of human conflicts and suffering both at the international level and in our own daily lives. It is the raging force behind our destruction of the forests, rivers, atmosphere, and all human oppression of the past and all that will come if we don't change.

Appreciation and Aware Care: When we change to the macrobiotic approach, our bodies are naturally able to begin a gradual process of dissolving internal physical hardness and inflexibility. Over time, normal, deep flexibility returns. This flexibility is much more than limberness only, it involves the internal organs and systems as well as joints and muscles.

The dissolving of the physical hardness and inflexibility also brings dissolvement of psychological inflexibility. However, this process takes time. Ki-Yō activities offer non-dietary possibilities for daily enhancement of this process of dissolving hardness. While dietary-induced physiological changes take place over time, Ki-Yō activities deal with the *right now* of psychological health.

Appreciation and Aware Care are essential aspects of Ki-Yō activities because they help us to move beyond the narrow focus on ourselves which creates tension and accumulation of tight energy in the mind. This tension and tightness holds us in a pattern of self-centered living that is characterized by insensitivity to our human family, beautiful earth and all of its life forms.

George Ohsawa often said that appreciation is essential to macrobiotic living. Appreciation is sensitive awareness, an expression of admiration, approval, or gratitude. When we feel life profoundly, there is in us the deeply active vibration of appreciation. It is not a sentimental feeling or intellectual practice, but more like a steady river that never stops. It is there, it flows. It is not an outward show for impressing people and manipulating them.

True appreciation is mostly anonymous. There is no "me" hiding behind it, nor is there any motive. It is a movement beyond the barriers of the hard self. In the act of such appreciation comes the dissolving of the burden of self-centered living. Appreciation is the natural response that arises from a deep sensitivity to the whole of life.

Does your life have beauty? I mean real, inward, breath-taking beauty. Inward beauty has nothing to do with where you live, money, or what kind of clothes you are able to afford. Are you in touch with the trees, children, and the moon, as well as the pain, sorrow, and ugliness? Can you embrace the ugly and uncomfortable as well the pleasurable and pretty? If so, you are touched by inward beauty and you are living with appreciation.

True Appreciation is endless. When it is there in your heart of hearts, you cannot bear to waste your life or anyone else's. Appreciation dissolves away built-up mental and emotional hardness. Like a stream that gradually dissolves boulders and pushes away the accumulation of debris, Appreciation gently acts upon the decades of built-up mental rigidity and insensitivity.

If the energy of one's life is primarily given to the building of one's own self-centered fortress of daily living, extreme psychological contraction and insensitivity intensify. Appreciation and Aware Care are activities that create outward-moving psychological energy when done in the right spirit. They assist with the macrobiotic process of changing our egotistical living into the art of living with a global mind and universal spirit.

True Appreciation and Aware Care involve the art of giving. They open us, empty us of the stagnation of self-centeredness and allow us wider receptivity to the universal abundance. Only that which is empty can truly receive. The internal energy that builds up as a result of self-centeredness, and the energy, created through Ki-Yō activities can be better understood in the following illustration:

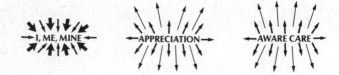

The modern I, me, mine way of living produces excessively contractive and constrictive mental energy. It creates physical and psychological tightness and tension which prevent the necessary elimination of energy from the body and mind. When we can't properly eliminate energy from the mind, psychological constipation develops.

Ki-Yō and other macrobiotic practices are meant to create within us a relaxed but strong quality of outward moving energy which allows us to openly and freely eliminate stagnation. Once this stagnation has been dissolved and we are maintaining a healthy body and mentality, we are able to consume, assimilate, and eliminate easily. Accumulations physically and psychologically are cleaned away. Our bodies and consciousness become clear and alert to any stagnation, dissolving it before it has the chance to build up and create problems.

Daily Activities of Appreciation and Aware Care: PEOPLE— Appreciating all people with whom we are sharing this life begins with active awareness of their presence. I am not writing about self-centered awareness of what they can do for me, but a fully alive awareness of *them*. Are you aware of people in the next car, in line behind you, or in the apartment below you? Do you have a feeling of care for them, or are you only concerned with what they think of you? Do you respond to people from your own self-centered addiction to their feedback and reassurance, or do you respond naturally because each person is your brother or sister? Watch yourself and find out.

Do you consume people, relationships and friendships in order to feed the roaring fire of your own ego, or are people free to be who they are when you are together? Are you another selfish member of the "mutual admiration society," killing others with kindness, or do you care about others enough to be frank and critical when necessary?

Are you living with a martyr mentality, thinking that you are being unselfish? Martyrs are full of resentment, anger and denial of feelings. They end up hating the people they have sacrificed themselves to. Is this your attitude toward people? Do you become so addicted to others that you are unable to contact your *own* feelings or find your *own* way?

When you are with others, be sensitively aware of them. Also become aware of your internal and external responses to others without condemning or judging these responses. Just watch. It doesn't take time or effort, and you will learn endlessly and honestly about your relationship to others.

Our day-to-day encounters with others provide the opportunity for healing through appreciation. Our words and behavior reveal a lot about our physical and mental condition. Is your behavior natural or artificial? Do you pretend to be open and full of smiles, hugs, and upbeat responses because others expect them from you, or are your responses springing from a deep inner sense of honesty and appreciation?

Upon entering a room or building, what is your response? Watch and see if you are at all aware of what is going on around you, or are you trapped within the walls of your own thoughts and demands? When entering a room, please send out your heartfelt and quiet feelings of peace and appreciation to all four directions, encompassing everyone present. In the same way, when you arise each morning, send your appreciation and peaceful intentions to the four directions, embracing every human being on earth.

If you do these very simple activities of Appreciation and Aware Care, you will find it very strange and difficult to hurt another, or use another.

NATURE—When we lose touch with nature, we lose touch with ourselves and every other human being. It is easy, living in big cities, to gradually remove ourselves physically and spiritually from nature, but I have also met many country-dwellers who have become numb to nature.

Everyone can have a love affair with nature rather than being divorced from it through insensitivity and lack of awareness. The more we awaken to our deep connection to nature the healthier we are. This connection involves more than an occasional canoe or camp trip. Awareness is where you are right now. Whether you reside in a fifty-story high rise or a fifty-acre plot of forest, you can express your appreciation of nature. Much more than a lover, doctor, priest, or politician, the natural environment sustains and supports your life.

Appreciation of the natural environment begins with our deep awareness of it. Wherever you are, when you look at the sky, the light of the sun spilling through leaves, the twists and textures of trees, and the endless colors everywhere, look with care. Look as though it is the first time, so that you really see and contact what is there.

The mind is so full of knowledge and assumptions about what we see, that we hardly ever see at all. Watch and see how much you miss because of the haze of words and conclusions that gets in the way of real seeing. Usually, when, we look at a tree, we don't really see that tree, but we are seeing our ideas, knowledge, and memory of the tree. We think, "There's an oak tree," "There's a pretty tree," or "I'd like to have that tree in my yard." Instead, see if you can look at the tree without the interference of words or thoughts, so that you are really contacting it. You will be amazed at the world that exists beyond the barrier of your thoughts and knowledge. Such openess and direct contact with the natural world brings deep healing.

Have you ever befriended a breeze, flower, or lawn of grass Does this sound silly or sentimental to you? I don't think it is, because only this kind of awareness and sensitivity can preserve and care for our earth. Only when we have this kind of care and appreciation for nature can we protect the land, skies, animals, and each other.

Do you thank the trees, plants, rocks, sky, sun, and water

for sustaining your life? Yes, actually thank *them*. It makes no sense to go to church to thank and praise God, but then go home and live in a way that is abusing nature. Please thank nature, praise nature, and care for nature. Please, everyday express your appreciation to the nature all around you by being deeply aware of it. Being so deeply aware is its own prayer.

Chapter 7
Nice Guys and Good Girls

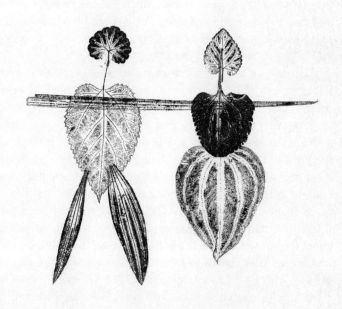

IKE TWO GOOD FRIENDS who care about each other deeply, let's be honest and share something of ourselves. Let's relax, take a deep breath, and be informal, as though we are sitting together under a tree or walking down a quiet forest path. There will be nothing to interrupt us, no cars or telephones, and no one else listening, just you and me.

Why not, if only for now, remove these masks that we have grown accustomed to? There, I hope you feel comfortable. Why do we wear them, anyway? Perhaps we have had them on for so long that we don't know how to live any other way. Here, though, you are my friend, and we feel relaxed, so it is not necessary to wear these false faces. We have real affection and care to know each other for who we really are.

You have probably heard of the "recovering alcoholic," right? Well, I am a recovering Nice Guy. There are millions of other Nice Guys and Good Girls out there in the world. I meet them everyday, and most of them don't even realize that they are unhappy and have so much hidden pain, confusion, and concealed anger gnawing at their souls. Masquerading as the Nice Guy or Good Girl is robbing their spirit of freedom and joy.

Many of us have become stagnant and bottled up without being aware of it. As a result, we harbor a sense of personal inertia, lack of direction, and inability to change habitual patterns or move away from addictive relationships and stifling situations. At an early age we learn to suck in our feelings and be nice, or risk being nothing. We learn to wear the nice face in public, but our rage, desolation, and discontent often emerge at home behind closed doors, like creatures from the inner murky lagoon of forgotten feelings and unresolved emotions. Spouses, lovers, mothers, fathers, and children know very well the full force of the internal turmoil and anger that screams from the mind and tongue of the person who has learned to be the Nice Guy or Good Girl.

At home, church, school, and work we learn to stuff our feelings, do what we are told, think as we are taught, and act with chronic dishonesty in order to "get along" in the world and "fit in" with the norm. We trade in our true selves for something of much less value. It is shocking how widespread and deep this suppression of ourselves exists—at the personal level as well as in society as a whole.

For most of my life I assumed that I had to cover up my true feelings in order to be liked. As a result, those feelings became strangely distant and inaccessible inside of me. Like interesting artifacts in a roped-off section of a museum, my feelings were there to observe and analyze, but I couldn't really contact them at the gut level. It was as if there were "Do Not Touch!" warnings all over my true feelings. I lost contact with my own truth and became a dishonest Nice Guy. Long after I had recovered from severe mental problems, this suppression and fear of expressing my true and honest feelings hounded me. For years I believed that I was the only one who lived with this kind of emotional repression. However, I have discovered that it is everywhere, and most people bear it like a jagged cyst in their soul. This cyst of suppressed feelings is constantly cutting them physically and spiritually. It almost killed me.

Many people are so out of touch with their own feelings and inner workings that they are especially confused when confronted by someone else's deep feelings and emotions. Often I felt a panic and painful awkwardness when witnessing someone else experiencing a wrenching emotional episode. I had a sense of suffocating in the other person's feelings and wanting to run away. Nice Guys and Good Girls often feel responsible for what other people are feeling, even strangers.

Nice Guys and Good Girls, being out of touch with what they are really feeling, easily assume the emotional states of those around them. If people around them are happy, or confused and disorderly, the Nice Guy or Good Girl is happy or confused and disorderly, too. For a Nice Guy or Good Girl, there is often no sense of where the emotional boundary between oneself and another begins or ends.

People who have experienced this know the kind of confusion and emotional imbalance that it brings. In my own life it has been tormenting. In grocery stores, if someone dropped and broke a jar, *my* face would turn red from embarrassment. At the checkout stand, *my* heart would race and *I* would break out in a cold sweat if the customer in front of me suddenly discovered that he didn't have enough money to pay for his purchase. I felt depressed and belittled for clerks whose chastisement by the boss I overheard while waiting to be served.

Because so many of us have a buried sense of low self-esteem, we unconsciously believe that our feelings are not worthwhile or that they simply don't count. As a result of this, we are often more in touch with the feelings of those around us than we are with our own. Everywhere I go I encounter people who are cut off from their own personal feelings but immersed in those of others.

Nice Guys and Good Girls desperately want to be liked. They have assumed, for a variety of reasons and experiences long ago buried from consciousness, that they are surely not likable as they really are. Instead, they learn to be what they think others want them to be. They become performers, actors and actresses, at the never-ending audition for the role of the most likable person at the office, home, party, school, or church. Most of the time they are completely unaware of this struggle to project a likable image. All the while they live with a sick, sinking feeling in their stomachs that comes from being untrue to themselves. This superficial image is a well-built dam that holds back a torrent of resentments, hurts, frustration, and anger. Nice Guys and Good Girls busy them-selves with incessant doing for others in harried hope of ac-quiring a sense of worth from the "Thank you," "Gee, you're a hard worker," and "What a good friend you are!" re-sponses elicited from those they try to please. Nice Guys and Good Girls are exhausted experts at trying to rescue and salvage other people's lives. They have an urgent habit of tearing away from themselves and storming into the lives of others. They are depressed when alone, and they feel anxious with time on their hands or nothing to do.

If they don't get involved in other people's lives, they get involved with something. Often it is a religion, a charity, the family, or a cause in which they bury themselves. Fortunately, for the many fund-raising activities that go on, there are countless Nice Guys and Good Girls who dutifully donate their time and money in exchange for the temporary ability to feel good about themselves. They would be embarrassed not to give something. People might think badly of them. I used to get panicky when I encountered people from charities standing in front of stores seeking donations from the entering and exiting customers. If I didn't have any cash on hand, I was horribly ashamed and did not go near the store. Nice Guys and Good Girls feel compelled to make offerings when confronted by donation seekers. They are intimidated by door-to-door sales people, too. They feel guilty and humiliated if they say "No."

Nice Guys and Good Girls actually become addicted to positive feedback from others. They need a regular "fix" of reassurance from others that they are ok, lovable, needed, and worthwhile, because they simply don't believe so themselves. Like any addict, they will go to great lengths to get their fix. Through overworking, perfectionism, taking on responsibilities they don't really want, and covering for others, typical Nice Guys and Good Girls allow themselves to be used, and they end up harboring enormous resentment as a result.

The fix of reassurance quickly evaporates. Before long we find ourselves out in the fast lane of people-pleasing again, while continuing to lose sight of ourselves. This kind of behavior is not done out of genuine care for others, but as a way of hiding from ourselves.

Keeping up the Nice Guy or Good Girl image drains vast quantities of personal energy. It makes us emotionally numb, inflexible, and anxious. We live with an unspoken fear that what we imagine to be our unlikable real selves will be accidentally exposed. We are truly out of touch with ourselves. We assume that whatever we are is worthless, and we certainly don't want others to find this out.

Nice Guys and Good Girls are not always shy, passive, or

withdrawn as one might expect. They can be loud, obnoxious life-of-the-party types, too, hiding their real selves behind a barrage of come-ons, false fronts, arrogance, jokes, and "I've got my act together" pronouncements. Many Good Girls do a careful job of projecting a "mother earth" image of strength and independence, when in reality they are hungering for care and affection, full of needs, and searching for ways of relieving the many hurts that have remained stuck inside for years. Nice Guys often present the image of the tough "jock" or playboy who is on top of the world. Deep down they are really sensitive men who yearn for freedom and release from emotional pain.

Our society encourages this kind of cover-up in a variety of ways. We learn to hide the honest fact, not to face the truth, but to project something false. When it comes to facing our own inner selves we believe that honesty is *not* the best policy. We assume that deep inside we stink, and we must do everything in our power to prevent our malodorous selves from being perceived. We do this from a very early age.

As a teen-ager I saturated myself with deodorants and colognes, and I was famous for my bulging pockets of stock-piled breath mints and chewing gum. I was certain that I would be the unfortunate bearer of the school's or party's worst body odor and bad breath. Exiting a restroom in a fog of air freshener, I was mortified to meet the eyes of someone entering, who, I was convinced, would forever associate me with whatever odors had escaped my efforts at complete obliteration. Oh, what a panic when I found myself trapped in a strange restroom with a broken toilet handle that made complete flushing impossible. Always there was someone knocking at the door desperate to relieve himself. I have never been a mechanically-minded person except in this predicament. If necessary, I would remain locked in there for as long as an hour, flushing and waiting, flushing and waiting, fumbling with the internal gismo until, at last, all evidence of my earthiness was on the way to its anonymous destiny. The poor soul at the door would just have to wait. I found it much easier to face his wrath, than to think of him facing my unfinished business.

In order to secure their image as the worthy and likable person, Nice Guys and Good Girls spend a lot of time manipulating people. The main focus of this manipulation is image management. I expended enormous amounts of time and energy trying to control people's image of me. Nice Guys and Good Girls unconsciously believe that they must do this or face the inevitable: people having their own perceptions which must, of course, be negative.

I even manipulated people who I didn't know and would never see again. I created for them the image of me that I wanted them to have. In stores, for example, I made sure that the clerk identified me as the exceptionally patient and understanding customer when all of the others were impatient and complaining. Although I was in a hurry, too, I would pretend to be patient, even when the clerk was being insufferably lax in attending to me. Upon approaching an expressway toll gate, I would make certain that I had the exact change. I didn't want the operator to be put out or inconvenienced by having to make change. He or she might not think well of me. In parking lots I would park and re-park my car so that the person in the car next to me wouldn't think, "He parked too damn close, I don't like him!" In restaurants, I had to be sure that the waitresses, busboys, and cashiers "knew" me. I wanted so badly to be their evening's most memorable customer. I left extravagant tips just to be sure.

Nice Guys and Good Girls look to the outside world for feedback that assures them they are worthwhile. They don't trust their own perceptions of themselves, only what is reflected back to them from the external world.

Nice Guys and Good Girls don't like to give their opinions until they have heard everyone else's. They wouldn't want to have the "wrong" opinion. They don't like to openly disagree or go against the popular point of view. They assume that they will be disliked or thought of as odd if they challenge the status quo.

Nice Guys and Good Girls have a very difficult time maintaining close relationships. Often, they want full control of the relationship for fear that it will otherwise develop in unexpected ways.

They have a horror of being vulnerable or letting anyone become too familiar with them. When they begin to have feelings about another that they don't understand, they usually find a way to terminate the relationship. For them, closeness is a very frightening experience, because they really feel that they aren't worth getting close to.

Because Nice Guys and Good Girls have stagnant channels of emotional elimination, emotional energy accumulates inside of them to the point where it must find devious and distorted ways of getting out. They often explode with feelings of rage that are totally out of proportion to the demands of a situation. This is usually quite shocking to everyone involved, because the Nice Guy or Good Girl normally does an astonishingly good job of keeping the outside image under tight control.

Deeply buried low self-esteem is the major common denominator fueling the behavior and attitudes of most Nice Guys and Good Girls. It is impossible for them to believe that someone would really want to be with them for the simple pleasure of their company.

The majority of people experiencing the Nice Guy/Good Girl patterns of behavior and emotional dysfunction are usually completely unaware of the fact that their way of living is hurting them, or that it is anything different from the way everyone else lives. There is a certain conspiracy of silence surrounding this suppression of ourselves. We act as if it is ridiculous to expect a life of personal freedom, spontaneity, and love of one's work. How about you, do you love your work? Are you doing everyday exactly what you love to do and want to do with your life? Macrobiotics has brought me to the understanding that anything less is ridiculous. What a joy and relief to know that I am free to live and create my own life regardless of whatever obstacles and challenges might be in front of me.

Nice Guys and Good Girls come from a wide variety of backgrounds, but most commonly they have emerged from emotionally suppressed childhoods where alcoholism, drug abuse, food addiction, workaholism, or religious fanaticism consumed at least one parent. They often have a history of sexual abuse or emotional neglect, and frequently they come from families that were abandoned by a parent or where one of the parents died before a strong relationship with the child was established. Many Nice Guys and Good Girls have come from backgrounds where, although chemical addiction, physical violence, and abandonment were not present, there was a family philosophy of emotional repression, rigid rules and regulations, and a quiet killing of individual creativity and freedom.

Commonly, Nice Guys and Good Girls come from divorced parents or otherwise extremely rocky parental relationships. They have learned to walk carefully on what they perceive to be a very thin ice of daily life. Nice Guys and Good Girls can come from what would be perceived as the "perfect" family. While these families are busy trying to be perfect, they usually have little time for open communication and deep understanding. Individuals from these families often grow up with assumptions, misunderstandings, and distorted, fixed self-images that will affect them the rest of their lives if not identified and discharged.

It is important that the behaviors and attitudes of the individuals involved in the Nice Guy/Good Girl patterns not be viewed as bad, or elicit feelings of guilt and shame. Before we have the freedom to change, we must be aware of what we are doing and feeling. If the awareness is not there, there is little one can do about it.

Many Nice Guys and Good Girls are attracted to macrobiotics. Anyone who comes to macrobiotics brings all of his or her prior conditioning into their new, and thus not yet well-understood practice of macrobiotics. Our past conditioning and patterns of behavior won't change overnight, even though we may be able to quickly change what is in the refrigerator or what goes into our mouths. It takes perseverance, courage, and honesty to cultivate a sense of self-reflection and awareness. Perhaps it is one of the most difficult things in life to become your own self-investigator, because we have spent so many years running from ourselves, hiding from ourselves, and hoping some expert can figure us out and come up with convenient answers. Those who become strong and clear in this self-investigation, shining up their lives in the process, discover the fluid reality that is of a totally different dimension than the meaningless path they once accepted as living.

Before we have dissolved our past conditioning, we often misuse macrobiotics or unconsciously misinterpret it as being supportive of our Nice Guy/Good Girl patterns of thinking and acting. Very often such individuals turn macrobiotics into another hiding place where they think they can attain some perfect image of themselves while covering up the practical truth. They try to live "macrobiotically," which to them may mean *never* being sick (i.e. pretending to always feel good and happy), and pretending not to eat "bad" foods. They want very much to be accepted by other macrobiotic people, especially macrobiotic teachers. There is a certain common paranoia among macrobiotic people who are still manifesting Nice Guy/Good Girl behavior. They live with a constant fear that someone across the room will be able to visually "diagnose" their internal organs and condition, and expose their most recent food binges. They don't want their good macrobiotic image to be spoiled.

They live in an uncomfortably split world of "proper" macrobiotic behavior and the secret world of their real behavior. True macrobiotics, however, is not this kind of thinking and behaving. Macrobiotics encourages people to open up, relax, feel comfortable with life, and become genuinely creative and sensitive.

Frequently, one encounters an attitude among macrobiotic

people that says it is absolutely unnecessary to do anything else but eat in order to completely change oneself. The individuals who believe this often end up frustrated when their obsession with food leaves them feeling empty and devoid of spiritual and emotional nourishment. I don't blame them when they leave this kind of narrow practice of macrobiotics. I would, too. Macrobiotics is not a prison. Some may feel that it is not necessary to share, discuss, or express their feelings or problems with others. Strangely, there are macrobiotic people who even think it is a sign of weakness to do so. This is, in my opinion, a holdover from the Nice Guy/Good Girl pattern of not expressing oneself and being out of touch with honest feelings. Such distorted belief has produced the notorious cold-hearted and stone-faced macrobiotic stereotype who proudly boasts of being unsentimental. Baloney! Be who you are.

There are many who would infuse macrobiotics with their own hang-ups and misunderstandings and then pass them on under the guise of "proper macrobiotic practice." Become your own leader and teacher, even if it is hard, even if you make many mistakes, even if you don't know where to begin. Don't believe anything anyone tells you, or anything you read. Find out for yourself.

Everything that has been suppressed inside of us needs to be discharged. All of the sorrow, anger, grief, and hurt is calling for release. Nice Guys and Good Girls often brush this off when I speak of it to them. They don't think it applies to them. How deeply they hide from themselves! Eventually each one of us will be faced with what we have suppressed for whatever reason. Macrobiotics will bring tremendous inward changes. Those who quit after only two months or two years of basic practice will never truly know what deep transformations can happen through macrobiotics. One thing for certain, if you don't want to change, don't start macrobiotics.

What about you, my friend? You have been patiently receiving my words. What about your inner life? Are you a Nice Guy or Good Girl? Are you hiding, pretending, nickel and diming your precious life away being what you really don't want to be and hating what you do? In order for you to become more in touch and aware of your beliefs, actions, and behavior, it may be helpful for you to participate in one of the many programs that are available throughout the country for emotionally stressed individuals. Nice Guys and Good Girls have found programs like Adult Children of Alcoholics (ACoA), Emotions Anonymous, and other programs dealing with the issues of "co-dependence," quite helpful as they progress with the marobiotic diet and lifestyle. As long as these programs help an individual find a way into personal freedom, I think they are wonderful. If, on the other hand, they become just another crutch for the individual, they are of little use, even detrimental to freedom. Check them out for yourself, and make your own decisions as to whether or not you want to pursue such a program.

Within macrobiotics there are many methods for self-discovery. Please find a good teacher who can lead you to yourself without creating dependence on his or her own authority and expertise. Contact the organizations listed in the Appendix for names and addresses of experienced macrobiotic teachers, and please seek out the happiest macrobiotic people in your area. Help each other to live peacefully and with natural dignity on this splendid earth.

My friend, I hope you hunger for truth. Develop an appetite for truth that never ends and is never satisfied. One can never get full of the truth. It is always there to be hungered for, always new. Shall we leave our masks off and just be here silently with each other for awhile?

Chapter 8

Making Peace With Your Parents

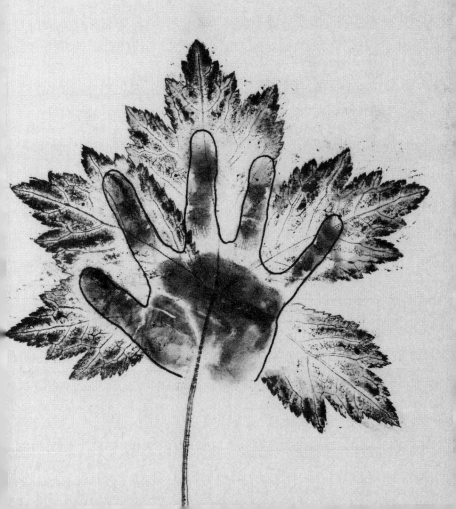

ACH ONE OF US SEEMS TO BE A TIME CAPSULE into which
has been deposited one's entire family history. The science
of genetics has demonstrated that the physical genes are
the means by which the physical characteristics of one generation are passed on to the next. However, what is passed
along from one family to the next doesn't stop at the physical
level. There is another aspect to gene transmission—a non-
physical one.

This invisible gene transmission contains two major facets.
I call them "psychological genes" and "spiritual genes."
Modern psychological theory supports, in its own way, the idea
of psychological genes. It has been established in the field of
psychology that patterns of family behavior are transmitted
through many generations. Children absorb their parents'
abilities, behaviors, views of life, and thought processes. Each
child adds his or her own idiosyncrasies and attitudes which
are then passed along when they have children.

The spiritual genes are similar to the psychological ones,
except that the spiritual genes pass on deeper and more un-
conscious aspects of ourselves, such as deep levels of happiness
and unhappiness, unresolved or buried emotional experiences,
and inner feelings. After many generations, a family estab-
lishes what I refer to as the "family spirit," which is the accumulated spiritual characteristics of an entire family. If one's
family has endured great suffering, if it has inflicted suffering on others throughout the years, or if it has been a happy
family and created many peaceful generations, this is held
within the memory of your spiritual genes. As a living member
of your family you have inherited some degree of its history.

A family is like an ever-sprouting plant from one generation to the next, appearing, growing, living in the world,
experiencing the multitude of ups and downs, maturing, and
finally withering away, leaving seeds behind to grow and go
through the cycle again. From one point of view it can be seen
as individual "plants" scattered through time, growing and
living independently, but from a much wider view it is more

truthfully one long and continuous movement of life, inseparable and indivisible. My family and I are one. Without any
one of them I would not be here. Through their lives they have
given rise to my own, and they still nurture me. As a living
member who has inherited the long history of his family, I
have now been passed the family flame to carry along. I can
affect the quality of this flame through my own life. Through
the way I live, I can quench any suffering, unhappiness, sickness, and disease that has been passed along to me in my
genes. I am now responsible for ending any sickness or turmoil
that lingers in the family spirit, because my family is now
me. Through the way I live, think, eat, and behave, I can pass
on a steady flame of health and happiness, or a terrible torch
of confusion, sickness, and unhappiness. I can heal myself and
my family in me, and I can also change the quality of the
physical, psychological, and spiritual genes that I will pass
along to the generations that follow me.

Many today wrongly assume that they have no personal
responsibility or power to change whatever they have inherited from their parents and ancestors. For example, there
are many who think that because their parents and grandparents suffered or died from hardening of the arteries or
diabetes, they are also destined to develop the same disease.
Others are afraid of getting cancer because, "It runs in the
family." Such thinking can only perpetuate pain and sickness
throughout a family's future. There are many family histories
of heart disease among people who are practicing macrobiotics, and many of the macrobiotic individuals were themselves in the early stages of the disease before finding
macrobiotics. However, they were able to reverse the
development of heart disease through eating macrobiotically.
By changing their health, they put an end to their inherited
history of heart disease. The mechanism is very clear: the
strengths and weaknesses of what we inherit can be made
stronger or weaker according to the way each individual lives
his or her own life. Most likely an individual from a family

with a tendency to develop a particular disease, *will* develop it if he or she continues to eat, think, and live according to the learned and inherited family traditions.

For me, developing an understanding and way of healing my family spirit continues to be the greatest of adventures. When we begin to heal ourselves, we start to break down resistance to the natural flow of energy within our bodies, minds, and spirits. When we establish physical health we are creating peace within our physical genes. When we have pychological health, peace comes to the psychological genes. Spiritual health brings a peaceful vibration to our spiritual genes.

One evening when I was about twenty-four years old, it suddenly struck me that I had never deeply expressed love for my parents. I realized just how distant I had been from my parents for so many years. There had never been any physical violence at home. My parents had definitely been more understanding than most of my friends' parents had been. There was, however, a subtle but deep lack of communication between us, especially between my father and me. In my mind, the differences between us became divisions, and I began to harbor enormous amounts of resentment, anger, and contempt. This added an extra burden to my already overwhelmed mind. I imagined that I was disliked at home and tolerated as the oddball of the children. I despised my parents for making me work hard around the house and yard. I thought I was being tortured for being different from my athletic brothers. I hardly knew my parents, and I was often afraid of them for no apparent reason.

Of course, I couldn't understand my parents at all when I was a boy and young adult. I used them and accused them. Never did I consider that they, too, were once children with parents who instilled in them various traits, and attitudes. My father was twelve when his father died, and my mother's mother died from tuberculosis one year after my mother's birth. Both of my parents lived through their difficult childhoods with a single parent.

Often people lose their parents long before they have actually died. Through lack of communication or plain ignorance, many people become distant from their parents. It becomes easier not to be with them because old patterns of behavior emerge, or old wounds ache again as incidents and feelings are remembered. As we grow up and move away from home, responsibilities of adult life mask the unresolved and incomplete nature of our relationships with our parents.

Frequently, when individuals have come to me for macrobiotic guidance, I have discovered that although dietary changes are almost always beneficial for them, they often have a much subtler problem at hand: the relationship with their parents. Sometimes just the mere mention of their parents' names is enough to bring tears or anger to their eyes. Some elderly individuals, as well as many other adults have sobbed uncontrollably after I began to inquire about their parents. Most of these people are highly successful in business or community affairs, and they are often looked up to by others. They wouldn't appear to have any great physical or psychological problems.

Among those who have been eating macrobiotic food, and getting good exercise and activity, there are some who remain deeply unhappy or who feel stuck in a rut of day-to-day living. In almost all of these cases I have perceived the presence of deep, underlying disturbances in the energy of the relationships with parents and ancestors.

As long as we are alive we are physically nurtured by the original quality of the father's sperm cell and the mother's egg cell. We have grown out of them, and from them we are influenced the whole of our lives. Mother and father are inextricable parts of us. They are in us. Without them we would have never been able to walk upon the land, see a sunset, or watch the stars. Although most people consider themselves to be separate or independent of their parents once they have moved away from them, we and our parents are, in fact, inseparable.

Many do not know or acknowledge that they are at war

with their parents. This war takes on a lot of different angles —physical, psychological and spiritual. As long as there is not peace with your parents, you are at war with yourself, too. Without having peace with your parents, how can you expect to have a peaceful relationship with a husband, wife, children, or friends? There are those who parade and protest in the name of peace, or to ask for respect from society, but when they put down their placards and return to their daily lives, are they themselves at peace with their own parents? How many are there who say they love God and attend church, but secretly hold on to anger and resentment toward their parents?

There have been many unhappy childhoods. Great numbers of children have been abused and neglected by their parents. Countless children have been bullied and belittled by their parents. Fathers have left home, mothers have deserted their families. Psychologists say that the majority of abused children become abusive adults. How about you? What has been and what is presently the relationship with *your* parents?

Please self-reflect about your relationship with your parents using the following questions as a guide:

1. When was the last time you told your parents you loved them?
2. Do you avoid being with your parents because you feel uncomfortable with them?
3. When you have conversations with others about your parents, what is the tone of your language?
4. How do you describe your parents to others?
5. If a parent is deceased, do you feel anger when remembering him or her?
6. When thinking about your parents, is it in terms of respect or thankfulness, or do you bear malice towards them?
7. Do you blame your parents for problems in your life now, or for your own negative behavior and emotional patterns?

8. Do you depend on your parents?
9. Do your parents have control over you financially or emotionally?
10. Do you struggle to live up to your parents' expectations even now as an adult?

One of the clearest signs that you are not at peace with someone is that you try to avoid that person, or when you accidentally encounter him or her you feel uncomfortable. A helpful way of contacting your feelings about your parents is to sit down and write a letter to them. Don't send the letter, just write it. Don't determine before you begin writing what you are going to say, just let the words flow into the pen and onto the paper, uninhibited. Do this several times over the period of a week, then look at what you have written. What do the letters show you? Are you at war or at peace with your parents?

Our parents have influenced us in so many ways, and this can be seen physically through external signs most visibly apparent in our faces. Of course, we already know that we inherit much of our physical characteristics from them, but other influences of our parents' reproductive cells can be seen as well. The many strengths and weaknesses of our parents are contained in their physical genes and imparted to us, and their psychological conditions, which are influenced by their physical health, are part of us, too.

Everyone's face can be divided into two sides (see illustration):

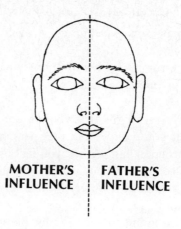

**MOTHER'S
INFLUENCE** **FATHER'S
INFLUENCE**

Take a picture of someone and make a copy of the print. Now cut both pictures in half. Put the two left sides or the two right sides together, and you will see that the person is very hard to recognize. The left and right sides of our face are different. This is because our parents, who influence our facial development, are different. When the basic structure of the face is forming embryologically, the right side is primarily influenced by the quality of the mother's egg cell and the left side by the father's sperm cell. The quality of these reproductive cells is essentially determined by the quality of the parents' blood. Therefore, the food, from which blood is made, is the foundation upon which our physical constitution is built.

If the reproductive cells of both parents are healthy and strong, then a generally more balanced appearance is imparted to the offspring's face. Extremely weak or unhealthy reproductive cells can impart an unclear or out-of-proportion look to facial features. If one parent was much healthier than the other, one side of the face will look strong with natural muscle tone, while the other will look loose and weak.

Besides showing the physical influence of the parents, the face reveals much about their psychological and spiritual influence as well. Observe the faces of those whose parents have been divorced or experienced many marital problems. You will notice some of the same signs of imbalance as those that are a result of unhealthy reproductive cells. The energy created by sadness and lack of communication between parents is imparted in subtle form to the children's eyes and face. On the faces of those whose parents separated early there is often a wide space between the eyes, indicating parental lack of to-getherness. Where one of the parents abandoned the family when the child was very young, it can often result in the child developing an eye that wanders out to the side rather than having a straight-ahead gaze. This shows that the nurturing energy of the parent has been very distant from the individu-al's life for a long time. These signs are not always readily apparent when one first begins to take notice of faces. They may exist in much subtler ways on the majority of faces that you observe.

It is important that this observation of faces should not be done as a way to make value judgments about people, nor does it have much to do with being "beautiful" or "ugly." Rather, it is a practical way of seeing how our parents in-fluence us, and realizing that we are inseparable from them no matter how far away they are or how much we have distanced ourselves from them emotionally. It gives us the opportunity to begin to understand what kinds of healthy or negative energies we acquire from our parents, and that unless we take personal measures to change our own daily lives, they can have numerous physical and spiritual repercussions.

Often I have counselled individuals who refused to make any moves toward making peace with their parents. They con-sidered the problem to be the parents' fault, and they pre-ferred to blame them for their own continued unhappiness as adults. Unless the parents changed, the individuals concluded, it would be futile to try to establish a sense of peace with them. These people are very unfortunate. They fail to find real peace of mind or life-long stability, even though they may become materially gratified or financially successful. More often than not, these are the people who drift from one quick relationship to the next, unable to get close to others, and wondering why they are single or always alone. They remain in a trap of feeling unloved and unwanted, never moving beyond their childish and painful search for immediate gratification and affection. They haven't learned to give love to others, because they are still waiting for it themselves. Or they greedily guard their affections, stingily rationing them to those who offer the most promise of a quick return on their affection investment. They are, without realizing it, passing along the same rejection and unhappiness that was received from their parents.

There is a variety of characteristics common to people who are not at peace with their parents. Among the most common ones I have observed are the following:

1. Lack of generosity. Calculating what one is giving and getting back. Stinginess.
2. False generosity. Giving excessively with the motive of buying people's friendship, affections, and attention. Manipulating people's image of yourself so that they will think you are so kind and helpful.
3. Hoarding things like furniture, clothes, antiques, etc.
4. Chronic suspicion of others' intentions.
5. Desire to control others and situations.
6. Belittling the opposite sex through your behavior and conversation, or belonging to a group or lifestyle that has a tendency to do this.

With any psychological or emotional sickness there is usually a concurrent physical condition and vice versa. Many women who hold anger, resentment, or negative memories associated with their parents, especially with their fathers (or other men), often suffer from the following physical conditions and symptoms: cysts and tumors of the breast, ovaries, uterus and kidneys, PMS, endometriosis, menstrual irregularity, and hormonal imbalances leading to excessive body hair and infertility. Men who hold negative emotions toward their mothers (or other women) regularly develop prostatitis, urinary tract problems, kidney stones, and symptoms associated with sexual function such as impotence, premature ejaculation, and hormonal imbalances such as lack of body hair and sexual confusion.

In addition, both sexes tend to develop problems in organs on the left side of their bodies when there are long-time unresolved emotional issues with their fathersi This especially influences diabetes, hypoglycemia, and other pancreatic disorders. With organs on the right side of the body, problems frequently arise when there are long-standing relationship imbalances with the mother. Among the physical conditions arising from this kind of stress to the body are liver, right lung, and ascending colon disorders. This is based on my own observations and interviews of hundreds of people during the last sixteen years. There are, of course, as many variations as there are individuals, but the patterns I have outlined above have become very clear. They are given so that you may further reflect upon the relationship with your own parents, and its influence on your own health and life.

Sometimes after discussing with individuals about the necessity of making peace with their parents, they conjure up a rosy picture in which they rush to tell their parents they love them and forgive them, and everything is suddenly wiped away and wonderful between them. It doesn't usually work that way. Like most of us, parents' lifelong habits and patterns of behavior can't be changed by someone else. *What one can change, though, is oneself, and therefore, any negative energies and influences that circulate inside of you.* It might always be that your parents will not express love to you, or apologize to you for any harm or abuse. They may never know how to acknowledge or even be aware of any negative influence they have had on you. They may never discover that they want to hug you or hold you. They may not know how to appreciate you or respect you. The change in your relationship with any one of them is going to have to come from inside of you, and you *can* let it happen. I have outlined the following steps for beginning to let this change happen inside of you:

1. Stop expecting anything from them, not in a resigned or resentful manner, but just cease having the expectation that somehow they will change. Many people *think* that they have done this, only to be upset and disappointed the next time they encounter their parents. You cannot change them, they are who they are.

2. Your parents are human beings with their own histories. Their patterns of thinking about themselves and life were heavily influenced by their parents. If you get the opportunity, ask them about their childhoods and how they were raised. Find out their observations and feelings. You may discover that they are suffering from their own unresolved feelings and conflicts relating back many years to their youth.

3. Start to learn and apply macrobiotic principles of living in such a way that you are best able to dissolve any physical hardness that has devleoped in your body from many years of consuming saturated fat, cholesterol, refined salt and sugar. Be patient. Your body will change gradually. Once hardness and physical inflexibility start to dissolve, you will be amazed at the emotional and psychological adaptability that comes to you. When you begin to change the quality of your blood through intelligent and consistent macrobiotic eating, the sticky and polluted internal condition that is the result of many years of unhealthy choices, changes to one where proper elimination and smooth function of organs return to your body. When smooth physical elimination is established, your ability to eliminate psychological and emotional stagnation improves as well. The resentments, grudges, memories and nightmares inside of you are much, much easier to understand and dissolve when your blood is clear of the debris from poor eating.

4. Play with a spirit of giving without wanting or expecting anything in return. To your friends, family, schoolmates, and strangers give of yourself in practical and helpful ways.

5. Every night before sleeping, wish your parents well from the depth of your heart, no matter what. Every morning, send out to them from your sensitive heart your wishes to them for a good day. If you do this, you will eventually be surprised at the depth of your true love for them.

Please play with these five steps in your own life. Do them sincerely even if you have no apparent problems. They are the most important steps I discovered for making peace with my own parents. With much affection I give them to you. Please make peace with your parents.

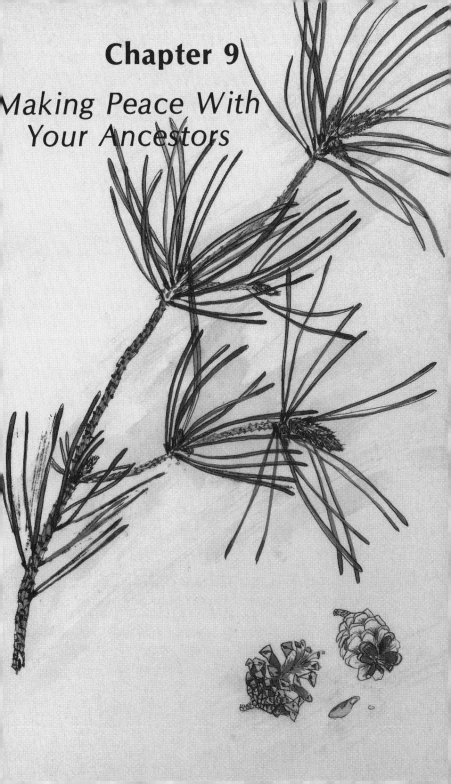

Chapter 9

Making Peace With Your Ancestors

I HAVE GIVEN MANY TALKS AND CLASSES over the years about macrobiotic subjects such as nutrition, cooking, home remedies, and cosmology, but none has captured the attention of an audience quite like the subject of ancestral healing. All eyes and ears are alert when this topic is being discussed, and the room becomes totally and strangely silent. It has been so whether I have been discussing ancestors with two or two hundred people. In this silence can be sensed strong presences and energies that fill the spaces around people. The atmosphere pulsates with expectation.

This unusual experience accompanies every one of my discussions of ancestral healing because of the urgent need for our help in the world of spirit. Audiences have given intense attention to this subject because each person feels something being touched deep inside. We all have ancestors, and we intuitively sense their appeals to us for love and assistance. We may have never thought about it before, or, if we have, it was always with the influence of TV and movies in our minds. We have been conditioned by the media to conjure up a world of spirits with images of the occult, seances, misty graveyards, and frightening stories. We have relegated the spirit world to the realm of the imagination, but my discussion of this topic has nothing to do with such silly notions and make-believe.

Ancestral healing is one of the most practical ways of establishing spiritual peace. Suffering in the spirit world can be greatly relieved by human intervention, bringing about tremendous healing within the entire family spirit that has been passed down through many generations. If you are completely sincere in your approach to ancestral healing, you will discover extraordinary changes happening in your life, for the healing of your ancestors is truly your own healing.

Your ancestors go back through countless generations and innumerable lives. It is hard to conceive of the thousands who have come before you and who have paved the way for your own life. To graphically grasp the extent of time and the energy of human life that has preceded you, look at the following chart:

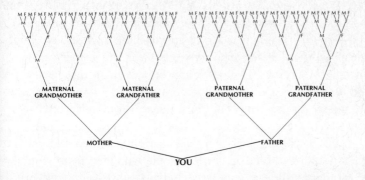

The number of ancestors continues to rapidly expand the farther back you go. Remove any one of them from the graph, and you can see that without that one life, yours would not have come into being. Each one of your ancestors has contributed something to the quality and characteristics of your life. Each one is part of you. What your ancestors thought, ate, believed, and felt have been passed along to you in a variety of subtle ways, and these influences emerge in your own daily life.

It would be, of course, impossible to know all of the details about your ancestors, but that is not what is important. It is only necessary to recognize the significant impact of these people on your own life. The spiritual strengths and weaknesses passed on to you by your ancestors are made weaker or stronger according to the way you live your own daily life. Family histories can be completely brightened and renewed by the development of a healthy quality in the present family members. If you put an end to greed, aggression, violence, grudges, dishonesty and self-centeredness in your own daily life, it can clear up the same qualities if they still linger in the family spirit. This lingering of negative energies in the family spirit comes about due to any unresolved or unhappy lives of ancestors. So, what you do in your own life not only heals you here and now, but also your past lives in the form of your ancestors, and your future lives in the form of the generations that will follow. If you don't pass along greed, pain, jealousy, anger, and sickness to your children, the history of their passing along in your family is put to an end.

There are two main ways of approaching ancestral healing. The first one, already mentioned, is the healing and transforming of oneself. The other approach is the direct pacification and assisting of deluded and suffering spirits of ancestors who are unable to pass smoothly into the world of spirit after death.

In the world of spirit there are many tormented and unhappy souls—soldiers killed in battle, people who died from painful or prolonged illness, oppressed Indians, slaves, inmates, prisoners, aborted babies, and many, many more. They linger and struggle within the hell of their own delusions, images, and thoughts. Just like someone who is asleep and having a nightmare, when we wake up struggling and deluded spirits, they are able to recover their true direction and be happy.

Each one of us has thousands of souls for whom we are directly connected because they are our more recent ancestors. The level of their spiritual health has an effect on us because the energy and consciousness of troubled spirits often attaches to the lives of present family members. Of course, not every spirit is a suffering one, but those who are, project their own delusion into the lives of the living.

One of the main purposes of religion used to be the assisting of souls during their birth and transition to the spirit world. This practice seems to have been almost totally lost among today's organized religious beliefs. Have we literally turned our backs on our own ancestors?

Oriental cultures have been particularly careful to remember and aid the spirits of ancestors, but this has certainly been part of other traditional religious practices, too. The Catholic Church, for example, celebrates the tradition of All Saints' Day (November 1), when a church member is required to attend Mass and is encouraged to pray for any suffering souls. Native Americans have the tradition of respect and remembrance of ancestors deeply woven into their religious rituals and daily lives. Early European cultures celebrated the sea-

sonal changes with song, prayer, and good wishes for de-
parted family members. Christian and other religious funeral
rites originated from the desire on the part of the living to
pay respects to and help a soul on its journey. This has often
been accomplished through singing, praying, and celebrations
involving offerings of food.

Most often in the West when a loved one dies, we consider
the relationship to be finished. After a period of grieving we
return to the daily routine and are encouraged by those
around us to gradually forget our sadness. We often speak of
death as a loss such as the often heard phrase, "When I lost
my . . . ." Death is not such a permanent loss. Our relationship with the deceased has simply changed.

In this physical world relationship depends on the senses.
We talk, touch, look, and listen in order to be in a relationship with someone. When that person dies, we are no longer
able to have a sensorial relationship, but we can establish a
spiritual one. There is no stronger relationship than that
which can be made between one who is here on the earth and
one who has been born into the spirit world. Because attraction and harmony of opposites is the underlying foundation of
this universe, the attraction between a physicalized human
being and one who is spiritualized is very intense, again not
on a sensorial level but at a much more refined and spiritual
one. This relationship can have many positive and negative
aspects. As we wake up deluded spirits who are caught in
their own nightmare, encouraging them on to their very
bright life in the spiritual world, we brighten our own spiritual qualities, too. If we don't wake them up, we can only
expect to be burdened with some form of their suffering
because of our inseparableness.

The modern way of thinking generally considers that the
physical and spiritual worlds are separate when in actuality
they are opposite but complementary aspects of one life.
The happiness or sadness of the spirit begins in *this* life. Our
spirit enters this physical world at the implantation of the
fertilized ovum in the uterus. At this moment, we arrive to

physicalize ourselves upon the earth after coming from the world of Infinity. During the time one spends in the mother's womb, nourishment comes from her blood which is created by the food she eats. Another kind of nourishment is imparted to us by the thoughts, feelings, and attitudes of both parents. In the womb we are living in a very small area, floating for nine months in a world of water. Our development there is determined by the quality of mother's blood which is delivered to us via the placenta and umbilical cord. This is the most important physical nourishment of our lives, for out of it our basic physical constitution is formed. This constitution becomes the foundation upon which one's entire life will be built. One's ability to think, act, respond, and view the world, will grow out of one's physical condition, including that of the brain and entire nervous system.

If the nourishment during this period is poor quality, the chances for impaired physical and mental development after birth are high. This has been made dramatically clear by the highly publicized effects of alcohol, drugs, tranquilizers, and malnourishment on newborn babies. The kinds of physical and mental harm done by polluted blood in the womb creates great difficulties once the injured baby leaves the quiet and safe environment of the womb's water world. Making the transition to the world of air outside the womb can be a traumatizing experience for such physically and mentally impaired babies. Often, even if there are no birth defects, babies have been severely weakened by improper diet and lifestyle practices during pregnancy. Many such babies have a difficult time being born, and frequently are premature or have to be taken by cesarean section. The need to keep these babies in specialized environments such as incubators and oxygen machines for weeks before they can go home, shows the tremendous difficulty of their adjustment to the demands of their birth into the air world. Each preceding stage of life prepares us for our birth into the next stage.

Once we are born into this world of air and begin to breathe, we are soon separated from the placenta and bloodstream of mother, although we will continue to depend on her blood outside the womb in a different form: her milk. Eventually, as the teeth emerge we start to take our food from the much larger environment of vegetables, grains, and other food products. During this time our physical and mental development is steadily taking place.

The body continues to grow and develop for many years because of our intake of nourishment. When the growth of the body reaches its limit in young adulthood, though, the consciousness experiences quickened development. As time passes and we further age, we begin to mature in our direction and thinking. We question the meaning of life, and our view of life broadens as we develop a more comprehensive understanding. Our appreciation for life deepens, and past mistakes or misunderstandings are reflected upon. As we mature in consciousness, our bodies naturally begin to weaken and lose the strong physical capabilities of our youth. All the time, though, we continue to take food and nourishment which vitalize our body, allowing for the continued development of our consciousness.

This process of developing consciousness takes place more or less naturally and smoothly according to the quality of nourishment we take, and the way we live our lives. Just as the nourishment in the mother's womb determined to a great extent our physical development, the nourishment we take in the air world determines the quality of the body which is the "placenta" feeding the developing consciousness. If this placenta is weak and polluted after decades of consuming saturated fat, cholesterol, chemicals, drugs, and so on, then the consciousness, which is fed by this placenta, cannot very strongly develop.

In traditional societies the elders were considered the most highly developed individuals. They were the most respected, and they were accorded great honor and high position within the society. Because of their developed consciousness, wisdom, and understanding, they were called upon to guide the course of the whole society. They were incredibly intuitive and able to determine how, when, and where they were to die. As their body grew weaker, they intuitively sensed the coming world of spirit and began to prepare for their birth into it. Because they had nourished themselves properly and lived a truly religious life, their birth into the next world went quite smoothly.

When we die, we leave this air world and are born into the much larger world of spirit. Just like birth from the womb into the air world, birth into the world of spirit can go smoothly or be extremely difficult. This is determined by the state of consciousness which has been developed during life. If the body has been fed excessive amounts of animal protein, chemicals, sugar, and junk food, the resultant quality of consciousness will be laden with heavy and chaotic vibrations which can be seen in ego-centered living. The consciousness that imagines, "I'm great," "I'm beautiful," "I'm powerful," "My possessions," will have tremendous difficulty leaving this world of air and being born into the world of spirit.

Every traditional religion has taught that what one does thinks, and experiences now will determine the quality of life in the spiritual world. Every traditional religion has had specific dietary laws, because the understanding of the effects of food on the development of the spirit used to be very clear.

When a person dies, their spirit (consciousness) leaves the body, and it can struggle to remain here in the air world if it is not fully developed and prepared for moving on. It doesn't want to leave if it has developed the consciousness of attachment, selfishness, and the illusion of a permanent identity. Like the baby born with physical birth defects, a deluded consciousness is born into the world of spirit with "spiritual birth defects," and it has a very hard time adapting to its new life. It may not even be aware that it has been born into the spirit world, so attached is it to its own worldly delusions and possessions. As if in a spirtual nightmare, it agonizes in its illusions trying to remain here. There are also "premature spiritual births" such as those caused by violent deaths. In such cases the consciousness is hurtled into the world of spirit long before it has had time to fully grow and develop. Such premature births to the spirit world happen when there are murders, suicide, abortion, and fatal accidents. The most severe spiritual birth problems, though, are caused by ego-centric living in this world.

A spirit which is unable to be born smoothly into the next world often attaches itself to familiar people, places, and things. Family members are the most common object of phy-sical attachment and, therefore, many generations can endure mental and emotional problems if the proper kind of spiritual healing is not done. Sometimes rooms or whole houses become the place of attachment as the spirit, caught in delusion and unable to free itself, hovers in turmoil in these places where it once lived. Antiques, furniture, and jewelry also become the focus of negative spiritual attachment. This energy of attach-ment is very, very strong. Take a look at your own attach-ments and see how strong they are. Can you easily let go of them? If not now, how much more difficult it will be when you die. It is essential that we dissolve our own hard ego in this life in order to develop a light and healthy consciousness.

Several years ago a friend was visiting my home and left me the gift of a small bowl with the suggestion that I make an offering of respect to my ancestors every day. I appre-ciated the gift, but I felt quite strange about making an offer-ing. At first I did nothing. I had always felt that making offerings to one's ancestors was fine for Orientals, perhaps, but it was not right for me. My background and traditions had never included care of, or understanding of, ancestors. I dismissed my friend's suggestion thinking, "I'm not into ancestor worship."

Then, when I was visiting my parents later, I off-handedly asked my mother if I could borrow some old pictures of my grandparents and other relatives to put on a wall in my apartment. I thought they would add an old-fashioned touch to a room I was redecorating. Mother agreed, and gave me an armful of faded photos from a trunk. One evening before

I had framed the pictures, I took them out to look them over. I arranged them on a shelf and then sat down on the floor to consider how they might best be displayed. The room was dark, and when I looked up at the pictures I suddenly closed my eyes and was met with an image of myself in the middle of a huge gathering of people. In the image I was kneeling on the ground, and they stood on either side of me as far as I could see. On both of my shoulders there came the sensation of pressure, and with my eyes still closed, I saw that the gentlemen on either side were resting their hands there. It was an incredibly firm and reassuring kind of pressure which I will never forget. I felt frightened and strangely comfortable all at the same time. This happened very quickly. When I opened my eyes I felt strange. "It was your wild imagination!" I thought. When I was sick I used to hear voices and have all sorts of wild imaginings. "No, this was different," I said to myself. There had been a definite presence in the room, and the pressure on both of my shoulders was undeniable.

For some inexplicable reason I looked at the pictures my mother had loaned to me and said, "Hello, I'm David, and I'm honored to be one of you," and then, "Thank you so much for your lives, because of you I am able to be·here." There was such a feeling of love and appreciation pouring from me. It is difficult to describe in words. "I promise, as a living member of our family, to live a life that is honest and sane. Through my life I will put to rest any sickness, suffering, and unhappiness that may still be lingering in you." Later I said, "Please know that your suffering in this world is over, and you can go on into your bright spiritual world. Let go of any attachments to this world." I felt as though a long-shut window had been opened, and crisp, fresh air was streaming in. I took a deep, relaxed breath and fell asleep. This was the beginning of the healing of my ancestors. It continues to be one of the most profound ways of creating peace that I have found through macrobiotics.

There is so much healing needed in the world of spirit.

I hope you can use the following suggestions for beginning your own ancestral healing process, and I encourage you to develop your own ways of bringing peace to the world of spirit, too.

There are many ways to approach ancestral healing. Some of them have come down to us from ancient traditions where care and healing of ancestors was a fact of life. Others can be quite personally devised by an individual for his or her own unique style. I would like to share with you the ones that I use most often and most successfully. Along with the food and cooking aspects of macrobiotic living, they have enriched my life in ways I never imagined possible.

The very first issue that must be addressed when beginning to explore the practice of ancestral healing is that of your physical and psychological health. Your own health will have a great effect on your capacity to help your ancestors. The stronger you are and the more energy that you have, the more you will be able to devote yourself to something beyond your own personal needs. It's hard to genuinely give when you are obsessed with your own aches and pains, and effective ancestral healing requires unconditional giving from your heart. In all areas of healing it is true: the less self-centered and self-serving you are, the stronger the healing power you can give. Egotistic ambition and desire destroy healing energy. They are blockages to the reception of universal energy which heals and renews.

Please consider healthy eating, exercise, and cooking according to macrobiotic principles of harmonious energetics. There is nothing I know of that can make you more sensitive. Give yourself plenty of time and the opportunity to learn and apply macrobiotic principles before you see long-term results of your effort. If you do this, you will someday understand why I have encouraged you so enthusiastically.

As a most practical and tangible way of beginning your practice of ancestral healing, I suggest that you create a place of respect and gratitude somewhere in your own living quarters. I call this the Family Memorial. Please choose a place that is quiet, if possible, and not easily disturbed or cluttered. This could be a mantle top, dresser top, or any other nice counter or table top. Take a sheet of paper and write across the top: "The Spirits of Ancestors." Then fold the paper into equal sides. On the left side write your mother's name and on the right side the name of your father. Directly above your mother's name write her mother's name slightly to the left and her father's name a little to the right. Do the same with your father's parents' names above his name (see the illustration below):

SPIRITS OF ANCESTORS

MOTHER	FATHER
MOTHER'S RELATIVES	FATHER'S RELATIVES
SISTERS	BROTHERS
OTHER FEMALES	OTHER MALES

Below each parent's name write the names of anyone associated with his or her side of the family who is suffering with psychological or physical illness, or who has suffered with such illness in the past. This should include uncles, aunts, cousins, and so on. Your brothers or any male friends should be placed under your father's name if you wish to spiritually console them. Sisters or female friends should be placed under mother's name for the same purpose. Anyone who you want to console spiritually can be included on this piece of paper.

Place this paper in some kind of frame or stand that will hold it upright so that you can see it when you come before your Family Memorial.

You can also place on your Family Memorial other helpful items. Especially good are a bowl of uncooked grain, a small bowl of natural sea salt, and another small bowl with purified water. Arrange them as shown in the illustration below.

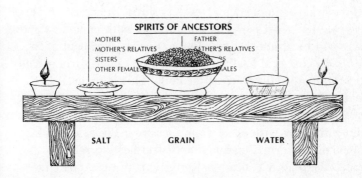

If you want, you may place two white candles and small evergreen plants on the memorial, too. You now have the basic traditional set-up of your Family Memorial. Please don't feel bound to this format. Your Family Memorial should come from your heart, that is most important. Feel free to improvise.

It is nice to arrange family pictures on your Memorial if you can obtain them, otherwise just the names will do. If there is someone who is sick or who has suffered before dying, please come to the memorial daily for about two months to offer your prayers or wishes of consolation to him or her. If there are no known sicknesses or sufferings, I suggest that you pay your respects and gratitude at the Family Memorial at least once a week, although it is really wonderful to do this every day.

Night time (before midnight) is the best time to help heal and console suffering spirits, but if you are just wanting to say "thank you" to your ancestors, then daytime is fine. Please change the salt, uncooked grain, and water at least once a week.

When expressing your love or prayers of consolation, it's not necessary to perform any particular ritual, although there are many that can be done. For beginning purposes it is only necessary to express yourself honestly and lovingly. A few minutes is sufficient. Keeping this practice very simple and clear is what is important. Never perform rituals or prayers that you don't feel perfectly comfortable with or understand. They will be absolutely meaningless, even detrimental, to successful ancestral healing. You may feel many strong emotions as you do this spiritual healing. This is natural. Let whatever you feel come to the surface to get released.

By preparing your Family Memorial you are reuniting yourself consciously with all of your ancestors. Please enjoy it. For further information about ancestral healing refer to the list of macrobiotic educational programs in the Appendix.

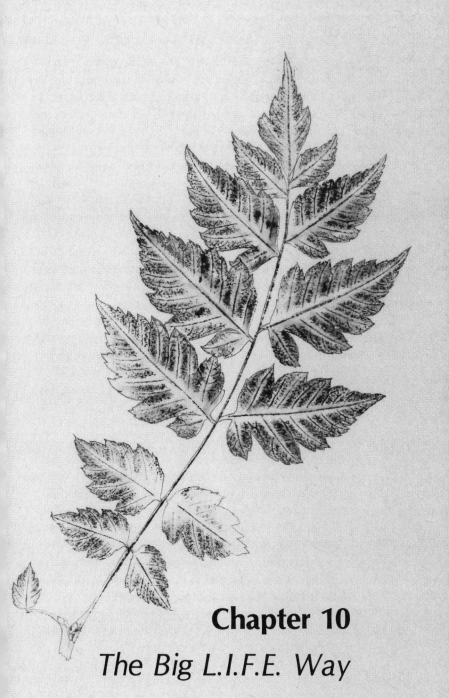

Chapter 10
The Big L.I.F.E. Way

A GAME IS FUN TO PLAY when you know the rules. The game is contained by the rules which define its boundaries, create its challenges, and make its requirements clear. The rules infuse dynamics into a game, and all participants agree to abide by them at the outset. Even spectators of a game must have a grasp of the rules if they are to fully appreciate and understand what they are observing.

When children create a spontaneous game, they begin by making up rules which will organize their play into easily perceived parameters of behavior. They decide together what they want to accomplish and how to go about it through making orderly rules. Without the laying down of the rules and the acceptance by all who want to play, there cannot be the fun and challenge that makes playing a game together so attractive. Even the subtlest and simplest of games has as its base a few common rules.

Everyone knows how easily the vitality of a game can be deflated by a disgruntled, losing player who, as his or her interest in the game begins to wane, tries to undermine the remainder of the game by humorously stretching or disregarding the agreed upon rules. Imagine the game where each one tries to play according to his own rules. Of course, total chaos would result. No one would enjoy such a disorderly blur of activity for long.

A game plan is specific to one particular game. Rarely can the rules of one be applied to another. Can you apply the rules of baseball to basketball? It would be absurd. Life itself is one immense game plan. If we know how to play it, it can be unbelievable fun. However, if we are ignorant of the whole game plan or if we apply the wrong rules altogether, life becomes a nightmare. Today it seems as if most people are struggling to use rules that make life a man-made *contest*, rather than learning the real Infinite game of life.

This contest in which so many people involve themselves I call "the little life contest." In this contest the word "life" stands for the following:

l = living	l = living
i = is	i = in
f = frustrating	f = fear
e = everyday	e = everyday

The real game of life, though, is so immense that I call it the Big L.I.F.E. Way:

L = Living	L = Life	L = Love
I = In	I = Is	I = Infinitely
F = Freedom	F = Fascinating	F = Flows
E = Everyday	E = Eternally	E = Everywhere

But the little life contest is the one most of us have been struggling to win ever since childhood when our education, religion, home, and culture began teaching us the rules. Every human being has learned these rules in one form or another, but for the sake of review let's go over the rules of the little life contest. They are as follows:

The Little Life Contest

Number of Contestants: Billions

Object of the Contest: Each contestant must battle against the forces of change to secure a permanent and separate identity for himself or herself through the acquisition of more power and possessions than the others.

How The Contest Goes:

1.   *PAWNS.*   Each contestant is a pawn of supposedly uncontrollable forces of fate. A pawn is moved backwards or forwards by the whims of destiny, and it is never known by the contestant when, where, or how the changes will occur.

2. *BLAME.*   No contestant is responsible for his or her own life. If he or she gets sick or becomes unhappy it is the fault of germs, heredity, or others' influence.

3. *CONFORMITY.*   A contestant depends on ideas, theories, authority, and fads for clues to the exact way he or she should live.

4. *ENEMIES.*   Every contestant must battle a legion of enemies on the path to becoming somebody and having a sucessful life. There are always the other contestants trying to get ahead, bacteria and viruses are crouching in every corner waiting to invade, and the ever-present chaotic forces of change are hiding in ambush around the next corner.

5. *SEPARATE AND DIVIDE.*   The contestants, in order to entrench and protect their positions in the contest, must separate and divide themselves from others through rigid beliefs, religious sectarianism, nationalism, race and other forms of separatism. The contestants must, at all costs, protect their own beliefs and possessions from those of others.

6. *MASQUERADE.*   Each contestant must play a variety of roles in order to get ahead in the contest. Each must protect one's own position while at the same time pretending to care about others and pretending to be considerate and helpful.

7. *ARROGANCE.*   Each contestant consumes as much as he or she wants, without respecting the order of nature and its dynamic laws as they apply to diet and health.

8. *CONFUSION AND FRUSTRATION.*   The contestant becomes confused, frustrated, and frightened when the man-made rules of this contest, while often providing the promised winnings, also bring the bitter bonus of sickness and lack of fulfillment. The contestant will feel free to shout, "Why me?," and complain constantly about misfortune.

Look around you. Everywhere people are struggling to win at this little life contest. How about you? Are these the same rules you fight to keep? The rules of the little life contest are taught everywhere—in schools, churches, homes, books, and on TV. Because of them, people have become confused and afraid. *Yes, they are the way to compete in this losing contest, but not the way to play the real game of life.*

In the little life contest, participants must battle to maintain their position and possessions, because in the blink of an eye they can be robbed of everything. There is always another contestant who is after what you have or conniving to take over your position and power. Stability and peace of mind are not part of the little life prize package. Disappointment and anxiety are the constant companions of contestants in the little life.

The rigid rules of the little life contest prevent people from playing the really big, unlimited game of life. The narrow limits of beliefs, dogma, political ideology, and national boundaries make the little life monotonous and cramped. The contestants are always at each others' throats. Life can never be fully played when we live within the narrow rules and limits of the little life that is being contested everywhere. Like gamblers at a twenty-four-hour-a-day casino, the contestants are aching for luck to turn in their direction.

Life is much bigger and more dynamic than the scrambling contestants of the little life can possibly imagine. It is sad to watch ourselves suffer because we are playing according to the wrong rules and game plan.

The real game of life goes on endlessly, and all we need to do is rediscover the principles of the Big L.I.F.E. Way and begin playing. The Big L.I.F.E. Way is a game, not a contest. Struggling and battling, while being a major part of the little life contest, have nothing to do with the Big L.I.F.E. Way. Let's learn its basic game plan.

The Big L.I.F.E. Way

Number of Players: Unlimited. (Each player enjoys teaching
more how to play the game, because the more players to
share the Big L.I.F.E., the more fun each player has as the
game's dynamics increase.)

Object of the Game: Endless play and enjoyment of life on
this earth through the understanding of the natural order
which is the foundation of life. There are no absolute
winners or losers, only players sharing the adventurous
game together.

How to Play

1. *RESPONSIBILITY.* Each player takes complete
responsibility for his or her own life physically, psychologically, and spiritually. No player blames others,
enemies, germs, or heredity for sickness or problems.
Responsibility means freedom.
2. *ORDER AND WHOLENESS.* Every player steadily
learns to perceive the natural order and wholeness that
is the essence of life. Through the continuous understanding of this order each player develops the capacity
to know why events happen, how sickness arises, why war
develops, and so on. Through the endless exploration of
this order and wholeness, each player begins to remember
where he or she has come from, where he or she is going, and the meaning of life.
3. *CHANGE.* A player clearly sees that everything is
changing, nothing is permanent. All struggling and battling for permanency is recognized as absurd and illusory.
It only leads to confusion and deep unhappiness. Non-
attachment is the natural outcome of understanding
change.
4. *YIN/YANG.* The player learns that change can be
viewed according to the natural Unifying Principle of Yin

and Yang. Through creatively playing with this principle, the player develops its applications to all domains of life.

5. *NON-CREDO.* Each player is aware of the danger of being enslaved by the blind acceptance of others' ideas, theories, and conclusions, as well as those of his own.

6. *ONE FAMILY, ONE WORLD.* The player is a member of one united human family, and does not separate from others through participation in rigid beliefs, religious exclusivity, nationalism or ethnocentrism. The player eliminates everything from daily life that divides him or her psychologically from the rest of humanity.

7. *FOOD.* Each player gains an understanding of the importance of the selection and preparation of food for the development of enduring physical well-being and human consciousness. This naturally leads to an understanding that goes beyond the modern nutritional knowledge of food and into the dynamics of the energetics and spirit of food.

We are all within this big game plan of life. No one is excluded. There are no rigid rules, only creative principles and the understanding of how life really changes in harmony and order. When you begin to know how the game of life goes on everywhere around you and in you, you can play along with it and have the greatest adventure.

Many people who eat macrobiotic food are still acting as if they are contestants in the little life. They think that macrobiotic food automatically makes them players of the Big L.I.F.E. Way. They are wrong. Food *is* a very essential aspect, but it doesn't change us mechanically. Some people have one foot in the little life contest and the other into macrobiotic food. They continue living by the rules of the little life long after changing their diet to whole grains, beans, and fresh vegetables. They become very healthy slaves of the little life, but not players of the Big L.I.F.E. To really play at it one has to bring the Big L.I.F.E. into one's thinking, attitude, and behavior.

If you are exclusive as you play, or use macrobiotics to gain prestige and personal power, guess what? You are still trapped in the little life. Your blood quality may be fantastic, you may never have a serious disease, but if you try to live macrobiotics as rigid rules and formulas, you cannot move beyond the limitations of the little life contest.

Will you play with me? If you are trapped there, step out of the confines of the little life and discover L.I.F.E.

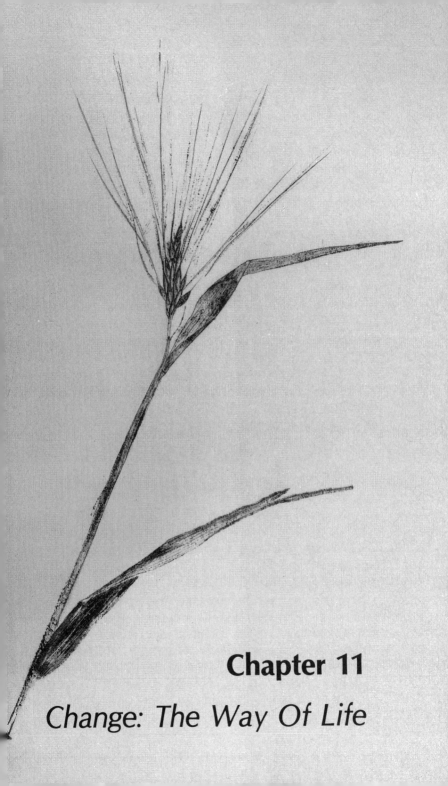

Chapter 11

Change: The Way Of Life

IMAGINE IF NOTHING CHANGED. Suppose the seasons suddenly stopped in the dead of winter and never moved on. What if the day were to stall forever at noon or the entire plant kingdom would remain locked for decades in the seed stage? Suppose your heart only contracted and your lungs could only expand. What if you could never sleep? Picture the kind of world we would have if everyone who had ever been born had not died. If the paralyzing sadness one has felt had never dissolved or the hysterical laughter at some silly joke had not subsided, could your life have continued?

For life to be, there must be change. Everywhere you look it is there, the constantly moving and changing song of life. *Where there is no change, there is no life.* Where natural change is impeded or resisted, life cannot go smoothly, and problems arise. When the natural changes within the ecological world are impeded, the balance of nature is upset. When the orderly physiological changes within the body are blocked or impaired, sickness begins; when a relationship between two people becomes dominated by one, stagnation and resentment build up: When the mind can't move from its obsession on something, mental disorder begins.

The understanding of the order of natural change in all domains of life is the essence of macrobiotics. To live consciously within the simple and dynamic order of nature is the daily aspiration of someone who practices macrobiotics fully. Macrobiotics is the art of understanding and applying the principles of the Order of the Universe in practical ways to live healthfully and cooperatively with nature and the rest of humanity so that we may all play together and enjoy life on this beautiful earth.

The Order of the Universe may sound rather grandiose and abstract, but as you explore its meaning and practicality, you will discover nothing but common sense. Living without knowledge of life's natural order is, of course, possible, but with a conscious grasp of it, life becomes far more interesting and enjoyable than one can imagine. Like a kid with a compass, you can always find your way and go any direction you wish with your life.

Everyone and everything is within this infinite Order of the Universe. It has been at the heart of every traditional religion. Everything is vivified by it, and all things and beings, are dissolved according to it. Whether you are aware of it or not, the infinite Order of the Universe embraces you, and its laws are universal.

We are all here sharing the same sun, moon, air, earth, and consciousness, but we have divided ourselves through beliefs, religions, geography, culture, and nationalities, and brought fragmentation to all aspects of life. Everywhere you look we have broken up life: in the professional world, in science, in medicine, in religion. They are all separate, fragmented parts of life. In the medical world we divide the body from the psyche, the eye from the ear, the heart from the liver. Everything is splintered and viewed separately from everything else. Such a way of thinking and viewing of the world can only lead to personal isolation and perceptions that all is chaotic and impossible to understand.

There is a different way of daily living. It is based on the fact that wholeness and order is the essence of life, not chaos and fragmentation. Macrobiotics encourages everyone to discover that life is a unitary movement of orderly and often predictable change. Rather than a rigid system of set formulas and beliefs, it uses simple natural principles as a *guide* through a free-spirited adventure of life. Once you learn the principles, you can do with them what you please. Macrobiotics suggests that by consciously applying the natural order to our daily lives, we become partners in sync with nature, rather than mere bystanders feeling alienated and jostled about by life.

When we ignore the Order of the Universe, we become uncertain and fearful. Disorder rules the day in subtle and insidious ways. We can't understand why events occur, how illness arises, or why our goals and dreams are met with so many obstacles. We scurry to give some semblance of order to our lives only to have illness and confusion disturbing our superficially imposed plan.

The natural order always responds justly and accurately to the choices we make. Sickness comes as a natural response to the way we have eaten and lived. Unhappiness is brought about by the way we think or the way we behave. There is nothing that happens without a cause in this universe, and there is no real injustice in this universe. Everything has a cause and purpose within the Order of the Universe.

The infinite Order of the Universe doesn't play favorites. Its laws apply the same to everyone, not just to people who eat macrobiotic food. No matter if you are a Christian, Jew, Hindu, Buddhist or atheist, male or female, heterosexual or homosexual, murderer or saint, you are treated equally by the Order of the Universe. Its order and justice touches all without exception. I have met dozens of ministers and holy nuns, saintly disciples and poor priests, social workers, sacrificers, wealthy families, and champion athletes who suffer from various forms of physical illness and mental disturbance because they have forgotten the wonderful Order of the Universe according to which everything comes into being, including sickness and health.

The simple understanding of the Order of the Universe was brought to the West in this century by George Ohsawa. Since Mr. Ohsawa and his students who came to America were all from Japan, many people have mistakenly assumed that macrobiotics is exclusively Oriental. The way of nature, the Order of the Universe, is wherever you are, whether you live in a temple in Tokyo or on a ranch by the Rio Grande.

George Ohsawa taught that the Order of the Universe could be viewed and understood in two ways, according to seven principles and twelve laws of change. We are experiencing them daily wherever we are. Everything proceeds according to them.

THE SEVEN DYNAMIC PRINCIPLES OF THE ORDER OF THE UNIVERSE

1. Everything is a differentiation of one Infinity.
2. Everything changes.
3. All antagonisms are complementary.

4. There is nothing identical.
5. What has a front (i.e., a visible side) has a back (i.e., an invisible side).
6. The bigger the front, the bigger the back.
7. What has a beginning has an end.

THE TWELVE CREATIVE LAWS OF CHANGE OF THE ORDER OF THE UNIVERSE

1. One Infinity manifests itself into complementary and antagonistic tendencies, yin and yang, in its endless change.
2. Yin and yang are manifested continuously from the eternal movement of one infinite universe.
3. Yin represents centrifugality. Yang represents centripetality. Yin and yang together produce energy and all phenomena.
4. Yin attracts yang. Yang attracts yin.
5. Yin repels yang. Yang repels yin.
6. Yin and yang combined in varying proportions produce different phenomena. The attraction and repulsion among phenomena is proportional to the difference of the yin and yang forces.
7. All phenomena are ephemeral, constantly changing their constitution of yin and yang forces; yin changes into yang, yang changes into yin.
8. Nothing is solely yin or solely yang. Everything is composed of both tendencies in varying degrees.
9. There is nothing neutral. Either yin or yang is in excess in every occurrence.
0. Large yin attracts small yin. Large yang attracts small yang.
1. Extreme yin produces yang, and extreme yang produces yin.
2. All physical manifestations are yang at the center, and yin at the surface.

This is simply another way of viewing life. If you are
patient and study its endless applications in your own life,
you will discover its fascinating truth and dynamics. Whatever phenomena, situation, or event that you scrutinize will
appear magically simple and orderly. I am reminded of some
lyrics from Leonard Bernstein's *Mass*:

> Sing God a simple song.
> God loves all simple things,
> For God is the simplest of all.

Macrobiotics is the singing of the simple song of the Order
of the Universe.

Everything is changing in order to be complete, harmonious, and alive. Everything attracts naturally that which
complements it, which is its opposite, and which makes it
whole. Macrobiotic philosophy uses the terms yin and yang as
adjectives to describe opposite tendencies that create mutual
attraction and wholeness through their interplay. Wholeness
is the result of yin and yang. Neither exists independently of
the other.

Examples Of Yin And Yang

	Yin	*Yang*
Attribute	Centrifugal Force	Centripetal Force
Tendency	Expansion	Contraction
Function	Diffusion	Fusion
	Dispersion	Assimilation
	Separation	Gathering
	Decomposition	Organization
Movement	More inactive, slower	More active, faster
Vibration	Shorter wave and higher frequency	Longer wave and shorter frequency
Direction	Ascent and vertical	Descent and horizontal
Position	More outward and peripheral	More inward and central
Weight	Lighter	Heavier
Temperature	Colder	Hotter
Light	Darker	Brighter
Humidity	Wetter	Drier
Density	Thinner	Thicker
Size	Larger	Smaller
Shape	More expansive and fragile	More contractive and harder
Form	Longer	Shorter
Texture	Softer	Harder
Atomic particle	Electron	Proton
Elements	N, O, P, Ca, etc.	H, C, Na, Mg, etc.
Environment	Vibration . . . Air . . .	Water . . . Earth
Climatic effects	Tropical climate	Colder climate
Biological	More vegetable quality	More animal quality
Sex	Female	Male
Organ structure	More hollow and expansive	More compacted and condensed

	Space	Time
Nerves	More peripheral, orthosympathetic	More central, parasympathetic
Attitude, emotion	More gentle, negative, defensive	More active, positive, aggressive
Work	More psychological and mental	More physical and social
Consciousness	More universal	More specific
Mental function	Dealing more with the future	Dealing more with the past
Culture	More spiritually oriented	More materially oriented
Dimension	Space	Time

As a practical example of the way the universal forces of yin and yang create change in our lives, let's take a look at the twenty-four-hour period we call a day. It is a gradual but constant movement between light (yang) and darkness (yin). Together they create one whole day, not in a flip-flop of opposites, but as a continuous transformation into each other. When the peak period of light is reached at midday, it is beginning to move towards darkness, and at the deepest part of the night there is the beginning of change back to light.

A flower can be viewed the same way, beginning as a hard, compact seed (yang), it gradually changes into a fully expanded blossom (yin) before changing into seeds again. The seasons, moon, life cycles of humans and animals, relationships, politics, history, astronomy, physiology, and any domain of life you choose to examine can be more easily and simply understood when you begin to study the common-sense philosophy of yin and yang.

When I started macrobiotics, I didn't know much about yin and yang and the Order of the Universe. When my first cooking teacher talked about the relationship of diet to health, I could easily understand, but when she discussed yin and yang I thought she was weird. Because I didn't personally understand it, I was prejudiced and extremely doubtful of the macro biotic philosophy at first. I thought, "The diet makes sense, but the philosophy is too far out and esoteric!" Even with this skepticism in my mind, though, I started cooking macrobiotically.

In the beginning of one's practice of macrobiotics it's not possible to have a detailed grasp of the macrobiotic principles of yin and yang. They have been outlined in this chapter in order to give you a glimpse of the philosophy underlying the practice of macrobiotics. When I began macrobiotics, I pretty much did what I was instructed to do, and followed recipes exactly and fanatically, although I now recommend beginners to *understand* and *question* what they do. I learned how to avoid "extremes" in my diet while preparing balanced macrobiotic meals. Later, I learned that to progress creatively, the study and application of the yin and yang principle would be the essential aspect of my development with macrobiotics. The study of it and free play with it taught me how to think macrobiotically for myself, and to steer my own life without unnecessary dependence on others.

The most important approach to macrobiotics which I have discovered is a relaxed and patient one. If you try to hurry your understanding of all aspects of macrobiotic philosophy, it will only serve to frustrate you, not guide you. As you explore the meaning and uses of the yin and yang philosophy in your own life, please have fun with it, challenge it, and test it. *Don't believe it. Find out for yourself.*

For further reading about yin and yang please refer to the Bibliography.

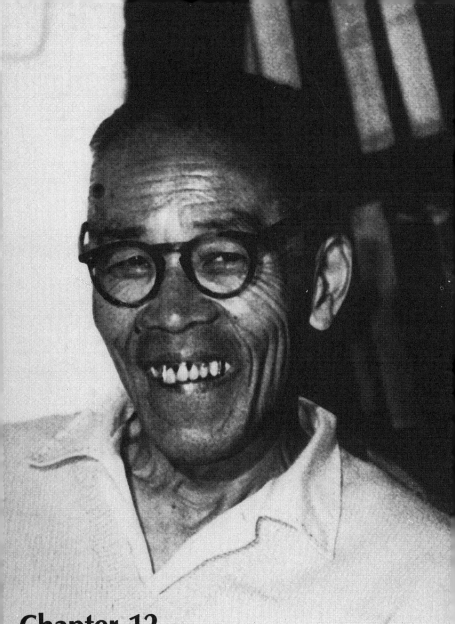

Chapter 12

*Dear George:
Open Letters To
George Ohsawa*

Georce Ohsawa was the father of modern macrobiotics. He died in 1966, six years before I began
macrobiotics. Over the years, through his books and
writings, he has had an indescribable impact on my life. At
first, I was put off by his words. He seemed harsh, demanding
and cold to me—who was very weak, wishy-washy, and used
to scheming and weaseling my way around life. When I read
something he wrote, though, there was a stirring underneath
my immediate dismissal of him as "fanatic." He seemed like
a friend, one who cared very much. Just like the order of
nature and its profound laws, his words scolded me, corrected
me, and always offered me the opportunity to change myself.
Hardly a day passes that I don't remember something that he
wrote, or think of him with affection and admiration.

This series of letters was started as a way to express my
gratitude to George Ohsawa and explore his teachings about
macrobiotics. They contain some of my ideas about a healthy
mind and emotional well-being. Please check the Bibliography
for books by George Ohsawa.

Free At Last

Dear George,

I can hardly write because of these tears, but I have to tell
you you were right—life *is* more wonderful than I ever imagined before. I'm finally out of that prison where I suffered
for twenty-nine years. I built that prison myself, didn't I?
Through my delusions and arrogance, I sentenced myself to
that miserable life.

I was scared when you shouted at me to jump to freedom
by jumping into the river of life, but I have done it, George,
and just like you said, I *can* swim and I *am* free. I tried to
escape from that prison by blaming others, lying, cheating,
and deceiving, but the bars of my prison became even stronger
Those days are over, and now that I am released from prison,
I can see skies beyond words, and the sunsets, George, the
sunsets! The moon, when it grows full, glows like the face of
an expectant mother. There are hundreds of birds in the trees,

and the trees are confidently rooted all around me, just begging
to be enjoyed. Their leaves change into indescribable colors in
the autumn. It is breathtaking.

I am like a kid at a carnival, George! This freedom is like
money burning a hole in my pocket. I can do with it whatever I want. Macrobiotics has set me free to live and play
and enjoy the earth. Sometimes I stand in the middle of
deserted roads taking huge volumes of air into my lungs and
exhaling like a kid blowing a balloon. It is such a relief to be
free! I wish you were here to be free with me, because I enjoy
the company of all that is free such as trees, backroads, and
birds. Nature is stunning in her freedom. Once when I was
walking down a road, I turned a corner and suddenly there
came a burst of birds from a bush. Their liberty astonished me,
and in an instant we were freedom friends.

Even in the city there is a showering of beauty. One night
I climbed to the top of a hill and was startled by the lights.
They were shimmering there below me as if stars had dropped
from the sky, and the city was treasure spilled aross the
horizon.

This freedom is so precious. I will never return to that
prison. Now I shout to others, "Jump, jump, jump into the
river of life!"

Jesus Said

Dear George,

The other day, after reading something you said about
Jesus, I remembered that he once said, "Unless you become
like a little child, you cannot enter the Kingdom of Heaven."

Many times I have thought about this saying. What did
Jesus mean when encouraging us to become like little children?
I started to watch children carefully, especially those who are
very young and still untouched by modern education and
cultural conditioning. I discovered, I think, what Jesus meant.

I have observed that little children share the following
characteristics:

1. Curiosity and Attention
2. Activity
3. Adaptability
4. Always learning
5. Honesty
6. Physical flexibility

Healthy little children are so curious and attentive to what is happening around them. Because their minds are not yet filled with preconceived ideas, they look freshly at life and absorb it. With their intense curiosity and attention, they are in a state of continuous learning and activity. For them there is so much of life to explore and enjoy. When was the last time you encountered a bored and uncurious child? Such a child would have to be one who is not feeling well.

Have you ever noticed that little children have no concept of enemies? Even when they bicker over toys and other possessions, their conflicts are usually quickly resolved when they are left to themselves. They learn that the more they cooperate, the more fun there is to share. Forgetting hurts easily, this morning's adversary becomes this afternoon's best friend again.

Healthy little children adapt so easily to different situations and environments. They are incredibly resilient. Hungry, cold, happy, sad, upset, or excited, young children express honestly through their words and actions what they are feeling. They don't know about lying yet.

Look at their fresh, new bodies. How flexible and internally clean they are! When they eat something chemicalized and junky, they naturally eliminate it through fever, diarrhea, or other similar symptoms.

A mentally or emotionally ill little child is rarely encountered. Only after they have entered school, or eaten chemicals and sugar for many years, can you find numerous cases of mental and emotional problems among children. Because little children are such recent arrivals from Infinity, they still maintain those qualities that we are naturally meant to possess

If properly and patiently done, macrobiotics can make us
like little children in spirit and attitude, and it certainly returns
youthful flexibility and health to our bodies. I have found
a very good gauge for checking whether one is getting healthier through macrobiotics. It seems more comprehensive than
visual diagnosis or the scrutinizing of one's daily excretions.
I tell people to watch and see if they are becoming more like
a little child in body, mind, and spirit, and enjoying their lives
in this Kingdom of Heaven.

Imitation

Dear George,

Michel Matsuda* told me that you abhored imitation of any
kind. Imitation is a subtle and pervasive kind of mental illness,
isn't it? It is everywhere today. Everyone seems so willing
and ready to do what some authority tells them to do. We are
conditioned to mechanically do whatever the doctors, psychologists, priests, teachers, and parents tell us. And for some
who come to macrobiotics, there is the secret hope that someone will tell them exactly what to do and give them the
perfect example to imitate.

Instead of thinking for themselves, there are those who go
around spouting answers from books, or constantly parroting
the pet concepts of their favorite teacher or counselor. I refer
to such individuals as "macro-babblers," and I have been one
of them myself. I'm sure you met plenty of them when you
were here, didn't you? They desperately want to be told
exactly what to think, how to look, where to go, what their
past has been and what their future holds.

George, can such an imitator ever be a truly healthy
person? A goal of a macrobiotic person should be the taking
of genuine responsibility for one's own life, right? That means
establishing a healthy body *and* a healthy mind. A macrobiotic

* Michel Matsuda, who was a student of George Ohsawa, now practices
acupuncture and lives with his family in Boston.

mind is one that frees itself from the conditioned dependence on authority and imitation. What someone else has said in the past may be true, but it has to become a living truth in my own life through my actual experience of it. Then it is mine, and I am not an imitator blindly following the example of others.

I am told that you lived and taught the macrobiotic spirit of *non-credo*, that is, the spirit of questioning, positive skepticism, and doubting in order to find out the truth. I agree with this spirit, George. It creates strong and enduring mental and emotional health. It is truly macrobiotic.

The Spiritual Ocean

Dear George,

We think we have to struggle in order to be happy. Once, I spent a whole week just watching myself and those around me struggle in a variety of ways. I saw the grasping for power, the battle to get ahead of others, jealousy, and the struggle to be recognized. I watched people hurt each other over the silliest, selfish things. Everywhere people were scrambling, scurrying, and trying to get somewhere faster or sooner than somebody else. There were poor people agonizing to be rich and the rich scheming to get richer. Even among some macrobiotic eaters and the spiritually inclined, there was the same greed, gossip, exclusivity, and battle to be better or separate from others.

Once when I was a boy, I was thrown into the ocean. I panicked, and because of my struggling, I started to drown. Miraculously, though, I relaxed and stopped fighting the water. The ocean buoyed me up to the surface where I could get air, see where I was, and swim to safety.

In our daily lives it is just the same. When we struggle psychologically and spiritually to be someone separate from others or higher than others, the huge spiritual ocean of life eventually sucks us under. We drown, struggling to hold power, possessions, and relationships.

The universe has a way of supporting and buoying up
ose who let go of egoistic struggling. When we have
ep understanding of the Order of the Universe, we know
at struggling is not necessary. People are afraid to stop
uggling. They imagine that life will pass them by if they
n't battle to be somebody. They don't sense that they are
ually drowning themselves. I can hear their cries for help
d see the desperation of their struggle, because one who has
own his own drowning immediately recognizes the sounds
d signals from others who are drowning.
When we stop struggling, we begin to take responsibility
 our own lives. When we stop struggling, we don't become
ssive and bored. We become full of energy to freely do
atever we dream. It has to be tested and found out for
eself.

A Balanced Mind

ar George,
There is a lot of discussion these days about the value of
ving a "balanced mind." It is a nice concept, but what does
 mean? Some minds are balanced as precariously as a tight-
pe walker trying to inch across the high wire to a secure
atform. The slightest jerk or jolt from life will cause such
mind to tumble. Others are balanced like the structural
sign of a skyscraper, only the most powerful and violent
sts of life can budge them. Some think that this kind of
ugh and immovable mind is a healthy one. In the same way
ey assume a rock-hard and muscle-bulging body is the sign
 a healthy body.
Such kinds of balance may be appropriate for a tightrope
lker or a skyscraper, but the balance needed by the human
nd is altogether different. It seems to me that the human
nd is balanced when it moves with the changing forces of
e and comes off balance or sick if it resists them. When
e's changing essence is perceived as the enemy against
ich we must gird ourselves and secure our position, mental

illness sets in. When I have had such an attitude about life, I *have* become like that tightrope walker, because I was fighting to maintain myself against the opposing extreme forces I created in my own mind.

True balance is not such a delicate position. It is not a static position at all. A balanced mind moves, changes, adapts, and harmonizes. It doesn't take a hard stand against life. A balanced mind is like a captain of a sailboat, reading the changes and directing the ship smoothly among the breezes.

Don't Get Healthy Too Fast

Dear George,

Sickness, sorrow, and suffering have been my best friends. I think of them fondly now as one might feel when remembering childhood companions. In all the years of my life there has been no book or person to give me what I have received from sickness and suffering.

I salute those who are sick and in sorrow. They have, more than all others, the potential for the greatest health and happiness. Through their own choices, they have made themselves miserable, and now if they learn to use macrobiotics as a guide they can build a wonderful life out of the ashes of their unhappiness.

In this astounding song of life, this ever-changing melody, the sick and suffering are the blessed of the blessed. When they become healthy and happy, they are forever grateful. No one is as grateful for food as the one who has been hungry; freedom is adored by the one who has been held captive; no one savors the face of a loved one more than he who has been long absent; the treasure of health is valued most by the one who has been so sick.

People who run from their sickness will never know health. Today it is easy for people to instantly stop symptoms through pills, but I encourage people to stay with their sickness for awhile, get to know it, understand it, and befriend it. Such friendship with sickness is the beginning of true health.

Intimate With the Infinite

Dear George,

My favorite definition of macrobiotics is one that you wrote. You said, "Macrobiotics is being on intimate terms with the Infinite." I found this to be such an interesting definition that I began to contemplate it everyday. What does it mean to be intimate? According to the dictionary, *intimate* is defined as "belonging to or characterizing one's deepest nature" or "marked by very close association, contact, or familiarity."

As a boy, I always longed to be intimate with God. My religion told me that because I belonged to its particular way, I was special to God, but I didn't *feel close* to God. Somehow I sensed that there was a way to know God in daily life. I could almost sense God, but when I strained my eyes and ears, I couldn't see or hear God. I felt sure that God was not something exclusive, because I had been taught that God was everywhere and in everything.

It wasn't until I read your book, George, that I found out how to become intimate with the Infinite. You showed me how perfectly simple God is. You gave me the keys to open the door: yin and yang. Now I see and hear God everywhere. This intimacy with the Infinite is the greatest love affair of all. Thank you, George.

Holding On and Letting Go

Dear George,

My favorite saying of yours is, "What you hold on to you will lose, what you give away is yours forever." It is natural, right? What we clutch and fight to keep inevitably slips away or is robbed. Now that I know everything changes, I can hardly keep from chuckling wherever I go. I have to remember to keep a straight face.

Everywhere people are so seriously hanging on to something: their youth, beauty, muscular body, money, diamonds, or health. They are really serious about it, George! It is a comedy, though. All that they hang on to is steadily changing and slipping away right before their eyes, and they can't seem to see it. Some of my macrobiotic friends hold on as tight as anyone else. They create their own rigid formula for living and call that macrobiotics. I can hear your guffaws right now, George. They are so surprised and sometimes disappointed to discover that everything *really does* change. They want macrobiotics to be a set pattern of living that never requires question or change.

Driving along the city streets, I often hear my mind singing out to everyone, "Let go and you'll have whatever you need." George, the universe wants to have such fun with us if we can only learn its glorious game.

Chapter 13
One Peaceful Day

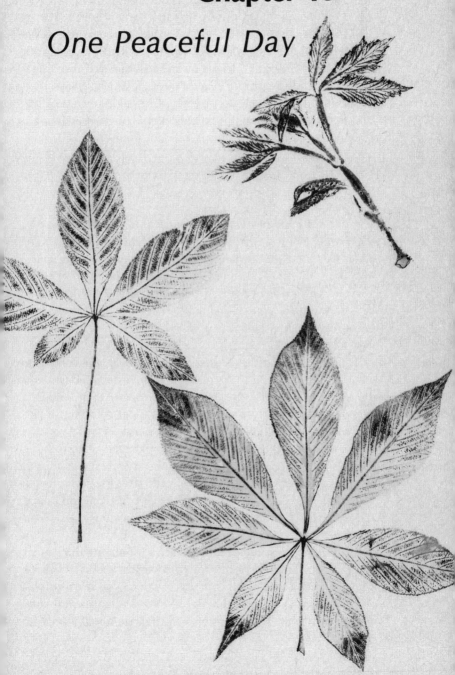

I AM WRITING THESE WORDS on the 13,972nd day of my life. For me, now, daily life is the most important issue, because what goes on here moment to moment has real meaning and deep significance. When we speak of living, of being fully alive, what do we mean? I discovered that for a long time after starting macrobiotics, I had just been theorizing about life, love, peace, and health. I came to the realization that mere theorizing and conceptualizing is not living at all. Life is the truth of what is actually going on inside and outside oneself. True living is not the living in stagnated ideas and memories, it is the actual moving *now*. It can't be described, you have to live it for yourself to find out.

What is daily living? If you can look at it directly, you will see that daily life has become a battlefield. Forget, for now, the battles being waged far away in the Middle East, Afghanistan, Central America and elsewhere. Simply look at your own daily life, for it is there you will find the truth. The majority of battles have nothing to do with guns and bombs. They are mostly unseen and subtle battles, and they destroy one's freedom and enjoyment of living on this earth with its vast magnificence.

There are the battles in the business world, the competition among religions, and the economic wars. In one's own daily life, there is the battle to be somebody better than the next person, the battle between who you are and who you think you should be, the inward tug-of-war between what you are doing with your life and what you would really like to be doing with it, and the eternal battle between your beliefs and those of another. There is the constant struggle to be loved, the conflicts and contradictions between what you think, say and do, and the internal war of concealed jealousy, envy and resentments.

Daily life can be the greatest teacher of all. Its movement brings everything necessary for discovering and establishing a healthy mind and happy life. Each day, if you learn to observe it, reveals the actual state of your present mental and emotional health. Psychologists can theorize about who you are, but to actually find out, you must be aware daily. Blood tests can't tell us much about our minds, and even if they could, they wouldn't be helpful for seeing who we are right now. For that we must, as Krishnamurti often reminded us, look into the mirror of our relationship with people, nature, and things everyday. We can know what we were last year or yesterday, and imagine what we might become tomorrow, but to see actually who we are, we must become conscious of what is happening right now without distortion. Your theories and beliefs can project comforting ideas and assumptions about who you are, but in the mirror of your daily life is the actual truth. That mirror doesn't lie.

Most of us think of our lives in terms of years. We predict that in so many years we will be this or that, or such and such dream will be realized at the end of a certain amount of time. What would it be like, though, if you approached life as just one day, because there lies its essence. One day is the seed from which your whole life blossoms.

One day is the concentrated version of your entire life. You can extrapolate from your observations of yourself during one day how you are choosing to live your whole life. Once, I was asked if I thought we could know in advance how we will feel at the time of death and in the consciousness following death. My response was as follows: if at the end of today, before you sleep, you can look back over your day and say, 'What a wonderful day it has been. I didn't waste it, and I have no regrets about it. I lived this day happily and with care," then you will probably feel the same way when you are dying. The period as we drift to sleep must be very much like the moment before dying. It is the death of the day, and the ending of your life in that day. It is really quite something if you look at it. You and your life come to an end at the end of each day.

Observe how you feel right before you sleep, and you will discover something essential. If, when looking back over today, you think, "I wasted this day doing things that I hated, working a meaningless job for more money, not speaking the

truth, not living happily or expressing my affection and love,"
then, you will probably end up with the same attitude and
regrets about your whole life. Look at the thoughts and feelings at the end of today, and contemplate what your life is
becoming.

The end of the day can be an extraordinary event. Instead
of carrying them over into your sleep and on into tomorrow,
you can put an end to the problems, grudges, and worries
that have built up during the day. Let them all go, drop them
easily, so that there is a sense of not holding on to anything
or anyone. Enter the end of your day with an empty mind
that is unburdened of the weight of self-centered living. Play
with this and watch what happens.

Like the end of the day, the morning is also quite reveal-
ing. If you have carried over the memories and problems of
yesterday, you can't be born freshly into today. You will be
stuck in yesterday, unable to meet the newness of today. If
you awake thinking, "Oh, no, not another day like yesterday!" or if you dread the coming responsibilities, appoint-
ments and activities, you will have great difficulty being born
into the new day. Morning is just like the birth into the
world of spirit after death. It has the quality of birth, the
entering into something new. If you struggle during your
birth into the new day, you are heading yourself into the same
kind of struggle and resistance when you will be born into
the world of spirit.

If you are constantly carrying over the regrets from yesterday, and always living in memories and knowledge of the past,
it is impossible to approach life anew or adapt to the challenge
and changes of today. Being reborn each morning with a mind
that says, "Here is a new day. It has never been before nor
will it come again. I am dedicated to learning from all that
happens today and to discover what it is to be truly alive.
Everything and everyone I encounter today is totally new.
With great curiosity and care I will look and listen as if for
the first time."

Many of us don't even realize it is a brand new day. Usually it is "the same old thing"—the same beliefs and stuck images of ourselves and others which we hold tight in our minds.

The essence of the macrobiotic view is "everything changes," and yet we can't live that truth when we remain mentally and emotionally quagmired in yesterday. Macrobiotics encourages everyone to move freely with the natural changes, but many seem to think this applies only to diet, physical health, and cooking with the seasons.

George Ohsawa is reported to have said to his macrobiotic students, "If everything is constantly changing—the cells of your body, seasons, atmosphere, and all that you see and hear, why aren't you changing your own mind and heart, too?" A mentally and emotionally healthy mind is a swift mind, one that is free to flow with the unending movement of daily life. If it gets stuck even for a moment, it begins to close and harden. A swift and open mind has no dams. Life moves through it uninhibited, and it is emptied continuously. Only such an empty, swift mind is capable of receiving the immediate, changing moment. Like a healthy digestive system, a healthy mind is one that consumes life, enjoys life, and easily eliminates what it takes in. Such an empty mind has a big appetite for life. If the mind gets jammed with uneliminated yesterdays, it loses its capacity to fully savor today.

The body's and mind's healing takes place through what one does *today*. Any healing is the result of what you start *now*, not what you plan to do next week or next year. In my experience and observation, people who have enduring mental and emotional well-being are those who are concerned with how they are actually living today. They are not hanging on to what they have been in the past or to what they hope to be in the future. Of course, practical planning for the future is necessary, but mentally and emotionally healthy people are primarily concerned with the reality of today.

College degrees, certification, seniority, and all of the other things we acquire to convince others that we are somebody, are meaningless compared to the fact of what you actually

are and do in the course of a day. The living truth can't be
found in what you achieved yesterday, but it is alive and well
in what you are doing now. Take an honest look at yourself.

Are you responsible for everything you do and think?
Are you even conscious of yourself at all, not self-obsessed,
but clearly aware of what you are actually doing from
moment to moment? Many today aim for some higher form
of consciousness before they've even become minimally
aware of what is right in front of them and inside themselves.
They shoot for the moon while their own little house remains
unknown to them. Our culture has educated us to strive for
tomorrow at the expense of living fully today. However, one
vibrant, fully lived, and happy day has more real impact on
life than a thousand fancifully projected and dreamt of
tomorrows.

It is easy to be a liar when we live in the fantasy of tomorrow or stay stagnated in yesterday's memories. Recently, I
came to realize what a liar I have been. I was convinced that
just believing in a peaceful life and world was enough. The
fact of the matter was, when I had the guts to own up to it,
that my daily life was actually anything but peaceful. I was
sharing a peaceful world dream, while my own daily life was
a nightmare of little wars. I had recovered from schizophrenia only to discover myself living on a more subtle
level of mental illness.

I had been eating macrobiotically for more than ten years,
I had healed the intense and overwhelming schizophrenia that
put me into hospitals, but now I found myself sharing the
common kind of mental illness that seems to quietly discolor
almost everyone's life. I was determined not to settle for half
healing. I was not satisfied with fitting into the socially accepted level of mental and emotional imbalance. Most who
met me perceived me to be healthy. They congratulated me
and respected me for overcoming my past illnesses. Yet I felt
troubled and uncomfortable because I could see that my day-
to-day living was filled with a multitude of subtle mental

illnesses and muted violence such as gossip, two-faced behavior and masked malicious intentions.

I was teaching health and peace but very covertly and unconsciously contributing confusion and sickness to the world of
my daily life. Hardly anyone would have called my behavior
sick, I wasn't doing anything different than anyone else.
Everywhere I looked and everywhere I went I could see
people behaving in the same way as I. My day had become
a dark comedy of contradictions.

It would have been easy to settle for a kind of mediocre
mental health, but I couldn't stop the healing urge inside of
me. The awareness that I was living so many lies grew with
such intensity that I began to feel embarrassed to go out in
public as a macrobiotic teacher. In front of the audiences that
came to hear me speak I felt hypocritical, but people admired
me. I could perform macrobiotic visual diagnosis quite accurately, even read people's thoughts, concoct all sorts of
useful emergency home remedies, and often predict futures
precisely.

In many macrobiotic people's minds, I had become the
quintessential macrobiotic teacher and counsellor, travelling
around the country, meeting hundreds of people, and hob-
nobbing with all the macrobiotic celebrities. I was envied.
I didn't have to beg to be on radio and TV shows anymore,
they pursued me. I began to feel like a fake in a carnival side-
show. On stage I was magic, the guy who knew the secrets
of natural healing and had healed himself. Off-stage I became arrogant and aloof. Up front I was patient, loving, and
thoughtful, but behind the scenes critical and condescending.
I wasn't macrobiotic at heart, only at the dinner table. I was
pretending. I had healthy blood, but I was unhappy. I could
see that after many years of macrobiotics, my real healing was
just beginning.

I could not sit back anymore and smugly say, "I'm healthy."
I had discovered that health is not a static point or an end to
be achieved. Like everything else, health is constantly chang-

ing. It is a daily process. I began to see that my old understanding of healing was transforming into a much deeper
one. My ulcers were long gone, the kidney problems had
healed, and the horrible fears and paranoia had disappeared.
Now there would be each day to heal and enjoy. This kind
of healing is never over. One can never say, "Finally, I am
finished healing my daily life," because each day is brand
new, and, therefore, unlike any other that has gone before.
I'm not suggesting that we see ourselves in a perpetual
state of sickness needing constant healing. What I am saying, though, is that everything that happens today is happening *now*, and in order to meet it one has to be incredibly
alert, aware and deeply honest. What happens today may be
similar to what has gone on in the past, but when we meet it
with a fresh mind, we are living within the reality of flowing
change.

I wanted to discover in a very basic and honest way the
truth of my daily life. What I had done before was over, what
I am doing today is the state of my health now. That is what
matters, that is where change is.

Macrobiotics had allowed me to become a normal functioning human being, and it had also awakened in me the energy
and sensitivity to see that "normal" meant settling for the
socially acceptable level of mental and emotional imbalance.
It wasn't enough to be normal, though. It meant remaining
with insidious sickness.

Honesty is a primary prerequisite for living one peaceful
day. Do you have it? Can you honestly and clearly observe
what goes on in your day from moment to moment and be
completely responsible for yourself within it? To be so deeply
honest and aware is one of the greatest things in life. Live one
day being quietly and completely honest with yourself and see
what happens. There are those who think that being honest
means being bluntly and harshly expressive of one's feelings
or caustically critical of others. There is a place for creative
criticism and open expression, but the honesty I am writing
about is much deeper than that. It is honesty inside oneself.

Such honesty is like a flame which eternally exposes all lies and hypocrisy It naturally burns away the dead wood of pretense and the tangles of contradictions, exposing the fertile soil out of which something new can grow. We are not used to this honesty, but when it comes, it brings such deep peace to the earth of one's daily life. Then, what was once your battlefield becomes your playground.

On this playground you can learn the answers to many interesting questions. What is the quality of your relationships? How do you view and treat your family, friends, neighbors, clerks, drivers, and strangers? What about your thinking? Is it divisive? Conflicting? Are there lies in what you say and do? Do you love what you do? Is your job good for others or only for your paycheck? Do you love anyone or anything at all, or do you merely depend on others and remain attached to them because of what you get back?

There, in daily life, one can learn the truth of oneself immediately. One day is the greatest teacher of all. From it you can learn what no book or consultation can give—the moving, changing truth of yourself and all of life around you.

Many people today are concerned with creating a healthy generation and new spiritual society for the future of humanity. Here and there we encounter prophets who predict a coming catharsis of disaster and nuclear holocaust. We are encouraged to get our health together, to meditate and pray for peace, and to pass the dream of peace on to our children. Isn't the real challenge, though, not merely to dream and pray for peace, which is really easy to do, but to *be peace today*? When one is intensely honest and in direct contact with one's own subtle battles and subdued secret violence, on a daily basis without guilt or attempting to force changes upon them, peace naturally arises. Play with it and see for yourself.

What today's society calls peace is actually just the lull between two wars, and its health is the anxious waiting period between two illnesses. We have come to settle for superficial and stagnating symptomatic responses to life's problems. We applaud nuclear treaties and at the same time continue the danger of nationalism that leads to war. We are excited and stimulated by the emotionalism and sentiment of peace rallies and ecumenical events, only to return home to daily routines where we unknowingly participate in the ways of thinking and believing which lead to division and conflict. We have become soppy and sleepy people.

What is important is how each one lives in daily life. If, in your daily life, you divide yourself from others through your beliefs, nationalism, way of eating, culture, thinking and other behavior, you are mentally and emotionally ill. You are contributing to the chaos and conflict of the world even though you may never leave your own backyard or throw a bomb. Where you are *is* the world.

> Bring yourself to life today,
> Moving, changing like the river's way,
> Freeing itself of yesterday's debris,
> By flowing now, it gets to the sea.
> For One Peaceful World we pray,
> And live its truth through One Peaceful Day.

Appendixes
The Spirit of Macrobiotics

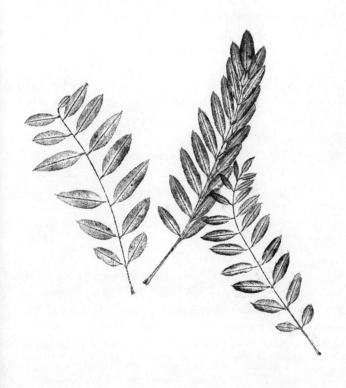

1. *Have Unconditional Faith in the Order of the Universe:*
    We should not let our emotions and our senses rule the
    destiny of our life. Let us live by our natural intuition,
    harmoniously working with the movement of the universe.

2. *Non-Credo:*   Do not imitate the theories and assumptions
    of others. Do not enslave your freedom with illusions and
    mysteries. Let us enjoy a spirit of non-credo, and let us
    seek endlessly, through our experience and understanding,
    what is clear and what is not, what is real and what is
    not.

3. *Be Our Own Master:*   As a human being, we must ex-
    ercise our own judgment. We may receive advice, sug-
    gestions and guidance, but it is we who should act as the
    master of our own destiny.

4. *We Are Ignorant:*   Being humble and modest by making
    ourselves the last, even to the extent that we are nothing,
    is the shortest way to have complete freedom of life.

5. *We Are What We Eat:*   We eat therefore we exist, we
    move, and we think. By changing what we eat, we change
    ourselves—body, mind and spirit—and also our society,
    culture, and civilization. Those who know this become
    masters of their life's destiny, and those who do not are
    slaves.

6. *Be Grateful for Difficulties:*   Hardships create understand-
    ing and appreciation. Difficulties are truly the cause of
    our happiness, and avoiding them is really the cause of
    our unhappiness. In order to be continually happy, we
    should continue to put ourselves in endless difficulties.

7. *Our Enemy Is Our Friend:*   The enemy who accuses and
    attacks us makes us cautious in action, deliberate in

thought, and strong in our abilities. We should be grateful to our enemies because they are antagonistic and complementary to us. They see, know, and have what we do not.

8. *The Last Become the First and the First Become the Last:* Yin is changing into yang, and yang is changing into yin endlessly. Therefore when we become high, we should remain modest, and when we become low, we should maintain our spirit of adventure. In this way we remain in harmony with the ever-changing universe.

9. *One Grain—Ten Thousand Grains:* Life is the process of receiving and giving, and the more we give the more we receive. Give, give, and endlessly give what is the most important, in order to make yourself and many thousands of people happy.

Standard Dietary Recommendations

The following are the standard dietary guidelines. The Standard Macrobiotic Diet, as outlined, can provide a starting point for establishment of good health for most individuals. It cannot be stressed enough that cooking classes presented by experienced macrobiotic teachers are very important and extremely helpful for improving one's ability to prepare delicious macrobiotic food. A listing of teachers and major macrobiotic centers is available from the organizations presented on the pages following this dietary outline. Learn how to be *relaxed* and *flexible* with this outline, not rigid.

Whole Cereal Grains: The principal food of almost every meal is whole grains. Cooked whole grains are preferable to flour products, as they are more nutritionally complete. Whole cereal grains and whole grain products include:

Regular Use	Occasional
Short-grain brown rice	Sweet brown rice
Medium-grain brown rice	*Mochi* (pounded sweet brown
Millet	rice)
Barley	Long-grain brown rice
Pearl barley	Whole-wheat noodless
Corn	*Udon* noodles
Whole oats	*Somen* noodles
Wheat berries	Unyeasted whole-wheat
Rye	or rye bread
Buckwheat	Rice cakes
	Cracked wheat, Bulgar
	Steel-cut oats, Rolled oats
	Corn grits, Corn meal, Rye
	flakes, Couscous

Soups: One or two cups of soup seasoned with *miso* or *tamari* soy sauce is recommended almost everyday. The flavor should be mild; not too salty and not too bland. Prepare soups with a variety of ingredients, changing them daily. Include a variety of seasonal vegetables, sea vegetables—especially *wakame* or *kombu*—and occasionally add grains and/or beans. Daily soups can include *genmai* (brown rice) miso, Hatcho (soybean) miso, *mugi* (barley) miso, or tamari soy sauce. *Kome* (rice), red, white and yellow miso may be used on occasion.

Vegetables: Daily meals include plenty of fresh vegetables prepared in a variety of ways, including steaming, boiling, baking, pressure-cooking or sautéing (with a small amount of sesame, corn, or other vegetable oil). In general, a smaller portion of vegetable intake may be eaten in the form of pickles or salad. Commercial mayonnaise and dressings should be avoided.

Green and White Leafy Vegetables for regular use include:

Bok choy   Carrot tops   Chinese cabbage
Collard greens *Daikon* greens Dandelion greens
Kale   Mustard greens   Parsley
Scallion   Turnip greens   Watercress
Leeks

Stem/Root Vegetables for regular use include:

Burdock   Carrots   *Daikon* (long white radish)
Dandelion root Lotus root   Onion
Radish   Rutabaga   *Jinenjo* (mountain potato)
Turnip   Parsnip

Ground Vegetables for regular use include:

Cauliflower   Acorn squash   Broccoli
Brussels sprouts Butternut squash Cabbage
Hubbard squash   Hokkaido pumpkin Pumpkin
Red cabbage   String beans

Vegetables for Occasional use include:

Celery   Chives   Coltsfoot
Cucumber   Endive   Escarole
Lambsquarters   Mushrooms   Romaine lettuce
Shiitake mushrooms Sprouts   Kohlrabi
Summer squash   Patty pan squash   Iceberg lettuce
Green peas   Snow peas   Snap beans
Wax or yellow beans Jerusalem artichoke Salsify
Swiss chard

Beans: A small portion (10 percent) of daily meals includes cooked beans. The most suitable beans may include:

Regular Use	Occasional Use
Azuki beans	Black-eyed peas
Chick-peas (Garbanzos)	Kidney beans
Black soybeans	Split peas
Lentils (green)	Navy beans
	Black turtle beans
	Great Northern beans
	Pinto beans
	Soybeans
	Whole dried peas
	Lima beans

Bean and Wheat Products: The following foods may be added to vegetable dishes or soups, as a substitute for bean dishes:

Tempeh: a pressed soybean cake, made from split soybeans, water and a special enzyme.

Seitan: wheat gluten, prepared from whole wheat flour.

Tofu: fresh soybean curd, made from soybeans and *nigari* (a natural sea-salt coagulant), and used in soups, vegetable dishes and dressings.

Dried tofu: soybean curd used in soups and vegetable dishes.

Natto: whole cooked soybeans, fermented with beneficial enzymes, served with whole grains, also in soups with vegetables.

Fu: dried, puffed and baked wheat gluten or seitan in soups or stews.

Sea Vegetables: These important foods are served in small quantities and comprise a small percent of regular intake. Sea vegetables are prepared in a variety of ways, for example in soup, with beans (*kombu* is especially recommended), or as side dishes. Sea-vegetable dishes may be flavored with a moderate amount of tamari soy sauce and brown-rice vinegar. Sea vegetables for regular use include:

Kombu: for soup stocks, as a side dish or condiment.

Wakame: in soups, especially miso soup, as a side dish or condiment.

Nori: as a garnish, condiment or used for rice balls, etc.

Hijiki: as a side dish.

Arame: as a side dish.

Dulse in soups: as a side-dish ingredient, or condiment.

Irish Moss: in soups or as aspic.

Agar-agar: for gelatin molds.

Mekabu: as a side dish.

Additional Foods: Once or twice a week, a small amount of fresh, white-meat fish or seafood may be enjoyed. Varieties include:

Flounder	Clams	Scallops
Halibut	Oysters	Shrimp
Sole	Red snapper	*Chirimen iriko*
Carp	Smelt	(very tiny dried fish)
Haddock	Herring (fresh)	*Iriko*
Trout	Cod	(small dried fish)

Roasted seeds and nuts, lightly salted with sea salt or seasoned with tamari soy sauce, may be enjoyed as snacks. Roasted seeds are used occasionally whereas roasted nuts are consumed much less often. These include:

Occasional: sesame seeds, sunflower seeds, pumpkin seeds.

Less Often: almonds, peanuts, pecans, walnuts.

It is preferable to minimize the use of nuts and nut butters as they are difficult to digest and are high in fats.

Other snacks may include rice cakes, popcorn, puffed grains, roasted beans and grains.

Desserts are best when sweetened with a high-quality sweetener, especially those made from grains, such as rice syrup, barley malt, and *amazake.* Dried fruit and fresh fruit may be eaten by those in good health. Fruit juice is not recommended as a regular beverage. Only locally grown fruits are recommended. Thus, if you live in a temperate zone, avoid tropical and semitropical fruit.

Sweets:

Sweet Vegetables	Sweeteners	Temperate-Climate Fruit
Cabbage	Rice syrup	Apples
Carrots	Barley malt	Strawberries
Daikon	Amazake	Cherries
Onions	Chestnuts	Blueberries
Parsnips	Apple juice	Watermelon
Pumpkin	Dried raisins	Cantaloupe
Squash	Apple cider	Peaches
	Dried local fruit	Plums
		Raspberries
		Pears
		Apricots
		Grapes

Beverages: Please use spring, well or purified (not distilled) water for teas. It is best to drink only when thirsty. Recommended beverages may include:

Regular Use	Occasional	Less Often
Bancha twig tea (*kukicha*)	Dandelion tea	Barley green tea
	Grain coffee	Local fruit juice
Bancha stem tea	*Kombu* tea	Beer
Roasted rice tea	*Mu* tea	Sake
Roasted barley tea	*Umeboshi* tea	Soymilk
Boiled water		Vegetable juices
Spring or well water		

Condiments: The following condiments are recommended for daily or special uses (Please use sparingly):

Tamari soy sauce: to be used mostly in cooking. Please refrain from using tamari soy sauce on rice or vegetables at the table.

Sesame-salt (*Gomashio*): 15 to 20 parts roasted sesame seeds to 1 part roasted sea salt. Wash and dry-roast seeds. Grind seeds together with sea salt in a small earthenware bowl called a *suribachi*, until about 2/3 of the seeds are crushed.

Roasted sea-vegetable powder: using either *wakame, kombu*, dulse or kelp. Roast sea vegetable in the oven until nearly charred (approximately 350°F. for 5 to 10 minutes) and crush in a *suribachi*.

Sesame-sea-vegetable powder: 1 to 6 parts sesame seeds to 1 part sea vegetable (*kombu, wakame, nori*, or *ao-nori* (green *nori*)). Prepare as you would sesame-salt.

Umeboshi plum: Plums which have been dried and pickled for over one year with sea salt are called *ume* (plum) *boshi* (dry) in Japanese. *Umeboshi* stimulates the appetite and digestion and aids in maintaining an alkaline blood quality.

Shiso leaves: are usually added to the plums to impart a reddish color and natural flavoring. *Shiso* leaves are known in English as beefsteak leaves.

Shio (salt) kombu: Soak 1 cup of *kombu* until soft and cut cut into 2″-square pieces. Add to 1/2 cup water and 1/2 cup tamari soy sauce, bring to a boil and simmer until the liquid evaporates. Cool and put in a covered jar to keep. One to two pieces may be used on occasion as needed.

Nori condiment: Place dried nori.or several sheets of fresh nori in approximately 1 cup of water and enough tamari soy sauce for a moderate salty taste. Simmer until most of the water cooks down to a thick paste.

Tekka: This condiment is made from minced burdock, lotus root, carrot, miso, sesame oil and ginger flavor. It can be made at home or bought ready made. Use sparingly due to its strong contracting nature.

Sauerkraut: Made from cabbage and sea salt, this can be eaten sparingly with a meal.

Other condiments which may be used occasionally are:

Takuan daikon pickles: a dried long pickle which can be taken in small amounts with or after a meal.

Vinegar: grain vinegar and *umeboshi* vinegar may be used moderately.

Ginger: may be used occasionally in a small volume as a garnish or flavoring in vegetable dishes, soups, pickled vegetables and especially in fish and seafood dishes.

Horseradish or grated fresh *daikon*: may be used occasionally as a garnish to aid digestion, especially served with fish and seafoods.

Pickles: including rice-bran pickles, salt-brine pickles or other naturally pickled vegetables; may be used in small amounts with or after meals.

Oil and Seasoning in Cooking: For cooking oil, we recommend that you use only high-quality, cold-pressed vegetable oil. Oil should be used in moderation for fried rice, fried noodles and sautéing vegetables. Generally two to three times a week is reasonable. Occasionally oil may be used for deep-frying grains, vegetables, fish and seafood.

Regular Use	Occasional	Less Often	Avoid
Dark sesame oil	Safflower oil	Olive oil	Commercially processed oils
Sesame oil	Sunflower oil		
Corn oil			Cottonseed oil
Mustard seed oil			Soybean oil
Canola oil			Peanut oil

Naturally processed, unrefined sea salt is preferable over other varieties. Miso (soy paste) and tamari soy sauce (both containing sea salt) may also be used as seasonings. Use only naturally processed, non-chemicalized varieties. In general, seasonings are used moderately. There are many, but those listed below are the most commonly used.

Regular	Occasional	Avoid
Miso	Oil	All commercial
Tamari	*Mirin*	seasonings
Tamari (*shoyu*)	Horseradish	All spices
soy sauce	Rice or other	
Unrefined white	grain vinegar	
or light grey	*Umeboshi* vinegar	
sea salt	*Umeboshi* paste	
Umeboshi plum		
Sauerkraut		
Ginger		

Recommended Daily Proportions

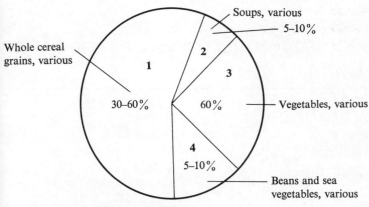

Plus occasional supplementary foods:
Fish and seafood, using less fatty varieties
Seasonal fruits, cooked, dried and fresh
Nuts and seeds, various
Natural nonaromatic and nonstimulant beverages, various
Natural processed seasonings and condiments, various

1. Whole Cereal Grains 2. Miso Soup
3. Vegetables 4. Beans & Sea Vegetables

1. Whole cereal grains are the principal food of almost every meal. These grains may be prepared in a variety of cooking methods; flour products, noodles and cracked grains, such as unyeasted whole-wheat breads, whole-wheat and buckwheat noodles, oatmeal, bulgar, cornmeal, and other cracked grains may be used to complement main servings of whole cereal grains.
2. One or two cups of miso soup or tamari-broth soup are usually eaten daily. The combination of vegetables, sea vegetables, and the occasional addition of beans and grains should change often.
3. Vegetables, served in various styles, comprise at least 25 to 30 percent of each meal. Vetegables are cooked by boiling, steaming, sautéing, baking, pressure-cooking, etc.; one-third or less may be eaten as raw, pressed salad or pickles.
4. Whole beans or their products, cooked together with sea vegetables, comprise 5 to 10 percent of a meal. (It is unnecessary to eat beans every day.) A variety of cooking methods may be used to prepare beans and sea vegetables.

Food to Reduce or Avoid For Better Health

ANIMAL PRODUCTS
Red meat (beef, lamb, pork)
Poultry
Wild game
Eggs

DAIRY FOODS
Cheese
Butter
Milk (buttermilk, skim milk)
Yogurt
Kefir

PROCESSED FOODS
Instant food
Canned food
Frozen food
Refined (white) flour
Polished (white) rice
Chewing gum

FOODS PROCESSED WITH:
Chemicals
Additives
Preservatives
Stabilizers

Ice cream
Cream
Sour cream
Whipped cream
Margarine

FISH
Red-meat or blueskinned
    fish such as:
Tuna (though raw
    tuna may be served
    occasionally with tamari
    soy sauce and a garnish of
    grated *daikon* or mustard)
Salmon
Sword fish
Blue fish

STIMULANTS
Spices (cayenne, cumin,
    etc.)
Herbs
Vinegar, except grain
    vinegar
Coffee
Alcohol
Commercially dyed teas
Stimulating aromatic teas
    (herb, mint, etc.)
Ginseng

VEGETABLES
Shepherd's purse
Sorrel
Avocado
Eggplant
Green & red peppers

Emulsifiers
Artificial coloring
Sprayed, dyed foods

SWEETENERS
Sugar (white, raw, brown,
    turbinado)
Honey
Molasses
Corn syrup
Saccharine and other
    artificial sweeteners
Fructose
Carob
Maple syrup
Chocolate

FATS
Lard or Shortening
Processed vegetable oils
Soy margarines

NUTS
Brazil
Cashew
Hazel
Pistachio

TROPICAL FRUITS-BEVERAGES
Artificial beverages (soda,
    cola, etc.)
Tropical or sub-tropical
    fruits:
Bananas
Coconut
Figs
Grapefruit

VEGETABLES	TROPICAL FRUIT-BEVERAGES
Asparagus	Kiwi
Bamboo shoots	Mangoes
Beets	Oranges
Curly dock	Papayas
Fennel	Prunes
Ferns	
Spinach	
Okra	
Purslane	
Green zucchini squash	
Tomato	
Potato	
Sweet potato	
Taro (albi)	
Plantain	
Yams	

Major Macrobiotic Organizations and Contacts

Please contact the following organizations for more information about macrobiotic classes and counselors:

Kushi Foundation
Box 568
Brookline Village,
   MA 02147
(617) 738–0045

Vega Macrobiotic Center
1511 Robinson Street
Oroville, CA 95965
(916) 533–7702

For information about lectures, seminars and personal study sessions with David Briscoe, or to schedule his *Personal Peace Workshops* in your area, please contact:

Personal Peace
2720 N. 46th St.
Kansas City, KS 66104

Bibliography

Aihara, Cornellia. *The Do of Cooking*. Chico, Calif.: George
Ohsawa Macrobiotic Foundation, 1972.
——. *The Calendar Cookbook*. Oroville, Calif.: George Ohsawa
Macrobiotic Foundation, 1979.
——. *Macrobiotic Kitchen: Key to Good Health*. Tokyo and
New York: Japan Publications, Inc., 1983.
Aihara, Herman. *Basic Macrobiotics*. Tokyo and New York:
Japan Publications, Inc., 1985.
——. *Kaleidescope: Macrobiotic Articles, Essays, and Lectures
1979–1985*. Oroville, Calif.: George Ohsawa Macrobiotic
Foundation, 1986.
——. *Learning From Salmon*. Chico, Calif.: George Ohsawa
Macrobiotic Foundation, 1980.
——. *Acid and Alkaline*. Oroville, Calif.: George Ohsawa
Macrobiotic Foundation, 1986.
Bloomfield, Harold H., M.D. *Making Peace With Your Parents*.
New York: Ballentine Books, 1983.
Chang, Stephan T., with Richard C. Miller. *The Book of
Internal Exercises*. San Francisco: Strawberry Hill Press,
1978.
Colbin, Annemarie. *Food and Healing*. New York: Ballentine
Books, 1986.
Esko, Edward and Wendy. *Macrobiotic Cooking For Everyone*.
Tokyo and New York: Japan Publications, Inc., 1980.
Esko, Wendy. *Introducing Macrobiotic Cooking*. Tokyo and
New York: Japan Publications, Inc., 1978.
Heidenry, Carolyn. *An Introduction to Macrobiotics*. Florence,
Italy: Alladin Press, 1984.
——. *Making the Transition to Macrobiotics*. Wayne, N. J.:
Avery Publishing Group, 1986.
Hoog, Deborah L. *Exploring Nature's Uncultivated Garden*.
Stroudsberg, Pa.: Rainbow Montage, 1987.
Ineson, John. *The Way of Life: Macrobiotics and the Spirit of
Christianity*. Tokyo and New York: Japan Publications, Inc.,
1986.

Jacobs, Barbara and Leonard. *Cooking with Seitan*. Tokyo and
New York: Japan Publications, Inc., 1986.

Jayakar, Pupil. *Krishnamurti: A Biography*. San Francisco:
Harper and Row, 1986.

Krishnamurti, J. *Krishnamurti to Himself: His Last Journal*.
San Francisco: Harper and Row, 1987.

——. *The Wholeness of Life*. San Francisco: Harper and Row,
1979.

——. *Beginnings of Learning*. San Francisco: Harper and Row,
1975.

——. *Education and the Significance of Life*. San Francisco:
Harper and Row, 1953.

Kushi, Aveline, with Alex Jack. *Aveline Kushi's Complete Guide
to Macrobiotic Cooking for Health, Harmony and Peace*. New
York: Warner Books, 1985.

Kushi, Aveline, with Wendy Esko. *The Changing Seasons
Macrobiotic Cookbook.* Wayne, N.J.: Avery Publishing Group,
1983.

Kushi, Michio. *The Book of Macrobiotics: The Universal Way
of Health, Happiness and Peace*. Tokyo and New York:
Japan Publications, Inc., 1986 (Rev. ed.).

——. *On The Greater View: Collected Thoughts and Ideas on
Macrobiotics and Humanity*. Wayne, N. J.: Avery Publishing Group, 1986.

——. *How to See Your Health: The Book of Oriental Diagnosis*. Tokyo and New York: Japan Publications, Inc.,
1980.

——. *Natural Healing Through Macrobiotics*. Tokyo and New
York: Japan Publications, Inc., 1978.

Kushi, Michio, with Alex Jack. *The Cancer Prevention Diet*.
New York: St. Martin's Press, 1983.

——. *Diet For A Strong Heart*. New York: St. Martin's Press,
1984.

——. *One Peaceful World*. New York: St. Martin's Press,
1986.

Kushi, Michio, with Stephen Blauer. *The Macrobiotic Way*.
Wayne, N. J.: Avery Publishing Group, 1985.

Lutyens, Mary. *Krishnamurti: The Years of Awakening*. New
York: Avon Books, 1976.

——. *Krishnamurti: The Years of Fulfillment*. San Francisco: Harper and Row, 1980.

Miller, Saul, with Joanne Miller. *Food For Thought: A New Look at Food and Behavior*. Englewood Cliffs, N. J.: Prentice-Hall, Inc., 1979.

Muramoto, Noboru. *Healing Ourselves*. New York: Avon Books, 1973.

——. *Natural Immunity: Insights on Diet and AIDS*. Oroville, Calif.: George Ohsawa Macrobiotic Foundation, 1988.

Ohsawa, George. *You Are All Sanpaku*. Edited by William Dufty, New York: University Books, 1965.

——. *Macrobiotics: The Way of Healing*. Chico, Calif.: George Ohsawa Macrobiotic Foundation, 1985.

——. *The Atomic Age and the Philosophy of the Far East*. Chico, Calif.: George Ohsawa Macrobiotic Foundation, 1977.

——. *The Unique Principle*. Chico, Calif.: George Ohsawa Macrobiotic Foundation, 1973.

——. *Jack and Mitie in the West*. Translated by Ken Burns, Oroville Calif.: George Ohsawa Macrobiotic Foundation, 1981.

——. *Gandhi—The Eternal Child*. Translated by Ken Burns, Oroville Calif.: George Ohsawa Macrobiotic Foundation, 1986.

——. *The Order of the Universe*. Translated by Jim Poggi, Oroville, Calif.: George Ohsawa Macrobiotic Foundation, 1986.

Ohsawa, Lima. *Macrobiotic Cuisine*. Tokyo and New York: Japan Publications, Inc., 1985.

Schuster, Mary I., *Creative Responses For Composition*. New York: Random House, 1973.

Stiskin, Nahum. *The Looking-Glass God: Shinto, Yin-Yang and a Cosmology for Today*. New York and Tokyo: Weatherhill, 1972.

Tara, William. *Macrobiotics and Human Behavior*. Tokyo and New York: Japan Publications, Inc., 1985.

Turner, Kristina. *The Self-Healing Cookbook*. Grass Valley, Calif.: Earthtones Press, 1987.